# THE MEANING OF AIDS

# STUDIES IN HEALTH AND HUMAN VALUES, VOLUME 1

Volumes in the Series

The Meaning of AIDS
*Edited by Eric T. Juengst and Barbara A. Koenig*
1989

Advance Directives in Medicine
*Edited by Chris Hackler, Ray Moseley, and
Dorothy E. Vawter*
1989

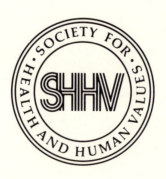

# THE MEANING OF AIDS

Implications for Medical Science, Clinical Practice, and Public Health Policy

Edited by Eric T. Juengst and Barbara A. Koenig

Studies in Health and Human Values

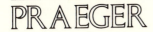

New York
Westport, Connecticut
London

**Library of Congress Cataloging-in-Publication Data**

The Meaning of AIDS : implications for medical science, clinical
    practice, and public health policy / edited by Eric T. Juengst and
    Barbara A. Koenig.
        p.    cm. — (Studies in health and human values)
        Bibliography: p.
        Includes index.
        ISBN 0-275-92646-X (alk. paper)
        1. AIDS (Disease).   2. AIDS (Disease)—Social aspects.   3. AIDS
    (Disease)—Psychological aspects.   4. AIDS (Disease)—Government
    policy.     I. Juengst, Eric T.   II. Koenig, Barbara A.   III. Series.
        [DNLM:   1. Acquired Immunodeficiency Syndrome.      WD 308 M483]
    RC606.A26M4      1989
    362.1'969792—dc19
    DNLM/DLC
    for Library of Congress           88-25464

Library of Congress Catalog Card Number: 88-25464
ISBN: 0-275-92646-X

First published in 1989

Praeger Publishers, One Madison Avenue, New York, NY 10010
An imprint of Greenwood Publishing Group, Inc.

Printed in the United States of America

The paper used in this book complies with the
Permanent Paper Standard issued by the National
Information Standards Organization (Z39.48-1984).

10 9 8 7 6 5 4 3 2

# CONTENTS

**Part Two: The Clinical Experience of AIDS**

**Part Three: AIDS and the Public Health**

# ABBREVIATIONS

| | |
|---|---|
| AIDS | acquired immunodeficiency syndrome |
| ARC | AIDS-related complex |
| ARV | AIDS-associated retrovirus |
| CDC | Centers for Disease Control |
| DNA | deoxyribonucleic acid |
| ELISA | ensyme-linked immunosorbent assay (test) |
| GRID | gay-related immune disorder |
| HBV | hepatitis B virus |
| HIV | human immunodeficiency virus |
| HTLV-I | human T-cell lymphotropic virus type I |
| HTLV-II | human T-cell lymphotropic virus type II |
| HTLV-III | human T-cell lymphotropic virus type III |
| ICU | intensive care unit |
| IDAV | immune deficiency-associated virus |
| IV | intravenous |
| KS | Kaposi's sarcoma |
| LAV | lymphadenopathy-associated virus |
| | lymphadenopathy/AIDS virus |
| | lymphadenopathy virus |

| | |
|---|---|
| NCI | National Cancer Institute |
| NIH | National Institutes of Health |
| RNA | ribonucleic acid |
| UCSF | University of California at San Francisco |

# FOREWORD
*Albert R. Jonsen*

AIDS (acquired immunodeficiency syndrome) is an inhumane disease. Its virus fastens almost unerringly on humans already affected by special social and physical vulnerability. It attacks the fetus, whose ability to defend itself is almost nonexistent. It attacks women in poverty, who are often the coerced sexual partners of infected drug users. It invades the bodies of the drug addicted, whose will to resist has already been captured by their habit. It massacres the population of male homosexuals, whose freedoms are already threatened by prejudice. AIDS seems to seek out as its victims the weakest and the already victimized.

Even its manner of attack is inhumane. It imprints on many the external stigmata of skin cancer. It sucks out strength, physical and immunological, and breath and mentation, leaving its victims husks of humanity. And on the way, it instills a fear not only of suffering and death, but of being the source of suffering and death to others, especially those with whom one has lived in intimacy and in love. Its inhumanity is near absolute, for it offers no chance of a fair fight; it bores in directly and vigorously to the very origin of the body's ability to defend itself. All disease is in some sense inhumane, enervating human hopes and powers and cutting off full lives. But most serious diseases have some touch of humanity; they attack high and low, weak and strong with a semblance of equality; they extend the courtesy of inviting the body to defend itself; they allow, at the end, a quiet surcease. But AIDS shows none of these humane qualities. It is prejudiced, utterly destructive, and coldly cruel in its killing.

This collection examines AIDS from the perspectives of the humanities. What have the humanities to do with this inhumane disease? First of all, one task of the humanities—history, philosophy, and literature—is to interpret the metaphor running through the first paragraphs of this preface. AIDS the disease, and human immunodeficiency virus (HIV) its agent, are not humans, with intellect, will, and emotions, and thus cannot literally be inhumane. This metaphor exchanges the effect for the cause. And this exchange, which can be found constantly in the writing and discussion about AIDS—and other diseases and disasters—is of great moment.

Science has created a language of objectivity, purged as far as possible of metaphor and innocent of historical reminiscence. This language, often mathematical, makes possible extraordinary mastery over nature because it enables human minds to focus on the phenomenon under examination and to communicate about it in precise terms. AIDS and HIV can, to a greater or lesser degree, be described in this language of objectivity: Epidemiology and virology and molecular biology speak in varying accents of that language. AIDS as a disease will be treated and prevented and defeated because these sciences have succeeded in discovering precisely what it is and how it behaves in nature.

Yet, at the same time that the sciences reach toward those discoveries, seeking the cause of AIDS, we live with the effects of AIDS. Some suffer with the disease itself or with the dread of its emergence within them. Some worry whether it can touch their lives or the lives of their intimates. Some write essays and books, devise programs and policies to treat it, contain it, prevent it. All those speak and write in human language, filled with metaphor, redolent of history, colored by emotion. They, as well as the scientists, will master this disease, if it can be mastered, because the pictures they paint in their own minds and in the minds of the public will direct public attention, mobilize public energy, modify public behavior, and generate public money.

The public language (if the term were understood less pejoratively, we might say the rhetoric) of AIDS is as important as the science. It is the task of the humanities to interpret and shape language. The critical analysis of forms of human communication and its logic as well as the creative production and appreciation of human expression have long been the work of historians, philosophers, artists, and critics. It is their duty to listen to the words people speak about AIDS and to ask whether those words are right and true: Do historical references reflect history? Is the logic sound that draws conclusions from premises and evolves generalizations from particulars? Is the moral reasoning about priorities with respect to social welfare and personal freedom consistent with the principles and values of our culture? Does literary style reflect or distort fact, elucidate or confuse meaning? These are questions the humanities can put to the public language about AIDS. Remember also that the scientists often speak this public language and often speak it as clumsily as do the uninitiated.

Take, for example, the frequent reference to AIDS as a "plague." That word comes with a history hardly known to most of its hearers or users. Yet it evokes powerful emotions that may fit the past better than the present. The secretary of the U.S. Department of Health and Human Services recently compared AIDS to the worst plagues of Europe. In numerical terms, the comparison is greatly exaggerated. Between 1347 and 1351, the Black Death destroyed 20 million people, one-third of Europe's population. By the end of the century, it had reduced that population by 50 percent. The best estimate of AIDS's devastation states that during the decade 1981–91, there will be a total of 180,000 deaths. Even though the numerical comparison is inaccurate, the realities are equally horrifying. The actual plagues of Europe and England in the sixteenth and seventeenth centuries have significant lessons about the obligations of physicians, the scapegoating of certain classes of persons, and the ease with which inferences are drawn between human catastrophe and divine retribution. Similarly, the epidemics of yellow fever, typhoid fever, and influenza in the nineteenth and twentieth centuries instruct us about the importance of public order and the utility, or lack thereof, of measures restricting individual freedom. These lessons are, mutatis mutandis, still valid in this modern epidemic. History alone can recall them correctly for our instruction. Philosophy, accustomed to reasoning about values and defining crucial terms, such as welfare, freedom, and rights, can guide discourse about the contemporary meaning of those lessons. Literature can reveal in vivid images the ravages not only of the disease, but of human folly responding to the disease. It reveals as well the victory of the spirit, the humility of the soul, and the courage of the heart that inevitably appear in the midst of the horrors of the epidemic. Camus's The Plague is an indispensible textbook for those who would see AIDS in human perspective.

The chapters in this volume are essays by humanists about the AIDS epidemic. These humanists—philosophers, historians, literary scholars, and others—have put their trained skills of recollection, perception, and analysis to the human experience of this disease. They have sought to clarify and correct definitions, to recall analogous incidents in our history, to draw values and principles out of the obscurity of emotion into the light of reason. These essays will not cure AIDS sufferers of the disease nor extinguish the disease from human society. The essays may, however, instruct us in how to live humanly and humanely while AIDS is among us.

# INTRODUCTION: THE MANY MEANINGS OF AIDS
*Eric T. Juengst and Barbara A. Koenig*

In 1985, the University of California at Berkeley sponsored an AIDS Awareness Week that was publicized by an odd poster. The poster featured a striking woodblock print of a snake coiled around an apple. The unexplained message of the poster proved controversial enough to gain the attention of local newspapers; the controversy centered on what the poster meant. Against the background of our culture's religious and moral traditions, the presence of a potent message in that image was unmistakable. The issue lay in deciding how to interpret that message and whether the message was justified. Did it merely express the deadly danger of AIDS and the seductiveness of the behaviors that put one at risk for it? Was it warning that those who risked AIDS also risked isolation from the (social) garden? Or was it suggesting that those dangerous, tempting behaviors were also immoral, and that AIDS was a kind of retribution for succumbing to them?[1]

Similar disputes over interpretation surround the meaning of AIDS itself. If we are to respond effectively to the epidemic, how should we understand AIDS? The cultural values and assumptions that color our interpretations of AIDS are often less obvious than the symbolism in the poster. Yet they lie in the background of our theories of scientific explanation and our efforts to contain the epidemic. AIDS's complex web of cultural meanings has the same practical significance as the poster's imagery: Left unarticulated they both can only generate misunderstanding, undermining our efforts to control the disease. The purpose of this volume is to uncover and analyze these cultural values and assumptions, using the interpretive perspectives of the humanities. Just as the discussion of the poster's design helped clarify its message, critically examining our vision of AIDS can help us see its implications and design our response accordingly.

Six different interpretations of AIDS seem particularly useful in introducing the chapters that follow. AIDS can be discussed as (1) a disease entity, (2) an illness experience, (3) a contagious infection, (4) a fatal affliction, (5) an epidemic disease, and (6) a challenge to individual liberty. Each interpretation has its own implications for our responses to the disease, and each can be loosely aligned with different professional, personal, and social points of view on the crisis. Moreover, these interpretations are analyzed in this volume from a wide range of disciplinary perspectives, including the humanities and the medical and social sciences. In spite of this diversity, however, the discussions that follow all share a striking feature. Consistently, the relations *among* the different interpretations are the key to their individual explication and assessment. Those concerned to understand AIDS, from whatever point of view, must recognize this interpretive complexity. The chapters in this volume suggest that effective and appropriate responses to AIDS—whether personal, clinical, professional, or political—will require a critical awareness of all those visions of AIDS, the links between them, and the implications we draw from them.

## A DISEASE ENTITY

One meaning of AIDS is the particular disease it names: a clinical entity described in terms of a distinctive pattern of signs, symptoms, and histories, and explained in terms of physiological processes traceable to specific causal agents. The discovery and description of that clinical pattern, the isolation and identification of its viral cause, and the unraveling of the disease process that links them are already considered a scientific triumph for medicine. These successes also provide a rich case for those interested in the complex dynamics of biomedical explanation.

For example, consider attempts of the Centers for Disease Control to define and distinguish acquired immunodeficiency syndrome (AIDS), AIDS-related complex (ARC), and human immunodeficiency virus (HIV) infection. The tensions are primarily conceptual, as traditional medical views of disease (as clinical syndromes or physiological disturbances or infections by pathogens) jostle for position within our scientific understanding of AIDS. Is this conceptual jostling an integral part of medical explanation or merely the lingering legacy of medicine's many competing etiological traditions? Similar questions about the role of other historical, cultural, and political influences in medical science are raised regularly in the AIDS story, from the early association of the AIDS immunodeficiency with "profound promiscuity" to the international disputes over the naming of the AIDS virus.

Of course, one reason that these "external" influences on science are prominent in the AIDS story is that our understanding of AIDS is not merely the product of scientific investigations of the disease. It also comes in large measure from our personal and social experiences of AIDS as an illness.

## AN ILLNESS EXPERIENCE

To take this perspective on AIDS is to ask what it means to have AIDS. Here, the important features of the disease are those that shape the experience of being ill with AIDS, such as the burdens of its devastating physical course and its stigmatized social status. To interpret these aspects of the disease one must look beyond discussions of AIDS within biomedicine to the fears, beliefs, and values that make the experience of AIDS problematic.

Besides being a particularly cruel illness, AIDS is multistigmatized: its lethality, its sexual mode of transmission, its association with socially "deviant" groups, and its physical stigmata can all serve to alienate and disenfranchise those who suffer from it.[2] How and why these characteristics of the illness create such intense social stigmata are cultural and psychological questions, the clues to which often lie in the language we use to discuss AIDS.

Both our scientific and experiential sources of knowledge about AIDS are explored in the chapters in Part One of this volume. Harold Varmus, Jana Armstrong, and Mary Ann Gardell Cutter examine aspects of the scientific explanation of AIDS, seeking to clarify the conceptual (and political) schemes that give medical meaning to the disease entity called AIDS. Judith Ross provides a bridge between scientific and social visions of AIDS by elaborating the metaphors that lace our public discourse. Then Joseph Cady and Kathryn Hunter and Julien Murphy explore the ways that cultural meaning and personal experience are reflected in language and literature about AIDS, drawing out the messages suggested by our responses to the disease. All these essays serve to show, in different ways, the extent to which our objective knowledge of AIDS as a disease and our subjective experience of AIDS as an illness are intertwined.

Parts Two and Three of the volume focus on two enterprises in which the close intertwining of the disease's biomedical and social meanings become particularly problematic: clinical practice and public policy-making.

## A CONTAGIOUS INFECTION

For health care professionals, one definitive feature of our understanding of AIDS is that it is infectious. This presses physicians to examine a theme within medicine's professional ethos that clinicians have had the luxury to neglect in the recent past—the fear of contracting a serious infection from one's patient. Professionals must consider the extent of their responsibilities to place themselves at risk of acquiring AIDS in the care of patients. In their chapters, Erich Loewy and Barbara Koenig and Molly Cooke explore historical and contemporary aspects of that theme, examining how the cultural meaning of AIDS shapes the medical profession's reaction to the AIDS crisis.

## A FATAL AFFLICTION

To the popular imagination AIDS signifies an inevitably lethal illness. This interpretation bears directly on much clinical decision making about patients ill with AIDS. What does it mean to say that one's patient is incurable? Physicians clearly have no obligation to provide futile treatment to their patients, and the ethics of forgoing life-sustaining treatments for terminal patients is much discussed. But when do treatments become futile, or patients terminal? For example, is the practice of establishing (on admission to the hospital) whether an AIDS patient should receive cardiopulmonary resuscitation ethically justifiable? From their respective medical and legal perspectives, Bernard Lo and Lawrence Nelson discuss the role that the special characteristics of AIDS patients should have in clinical decision making about their care. Similarly, Ray Moseley examines the question of how intensive care technologies and services should be allocated between AIDS patients and other critically ill patients. Of course, these problems are encountered to some degree in the care of any seriously ill patient. However, the prism provided by AIDS is particularly useful in revealing how clinical "facts" about prognosis may be influenced by value judgments about patients with undesirable social characteristics.

The transmissibility and lethality of AIDS also underscore questions about physicians' duties to curb the spread of the disease. In his essay, William Winslade addresses the conflict between clinicians' duties to protect the confidentiality of patients under their direct care versus their responsibility to warn third parties—for example, the sexual partners of an HIV-infected patient—that they are at risk of contracting AIDS. In the past, discussions of this issue have often been swayed by social views of personal culpability for disease. Professional duties have been held to depend dramatically on whether one's patients were classified as "incorrigible sources of infection" who brought disease upon themselves or merely "innocent victims" who paid the price of someone else's reckless behavior. By echoing that language, current discussions of the physician's duty to protect third parties from AIDS nicely illustrates the ways in which subtle social evaluations of patients can shape professional discourse.

## AN EPIDEMIC DISEASE

For public health officials the consequences of the spread of AIDS throughout the population are the primary concern: AIDS is for them first and foremost a serious epidemic disease. In this century, public health measures have accomplished impressive goals in the control of many communicable diseases; it is natural to contemplate pursuing the same policies with respect to AIDS. However, AIDS has confounding features that force us to reassess some traditional infection control strategies. Does premarital screening for AIDS make sense, for example, in a disease with multiple routes of transmission and a significant detection delay? Or is this approach merely a vestige of historical approaches that separated disease sufferers into categories of the guilty and the innocent? The third part of the volume addresses the issues raised by our understanding of AIDS as a major public health problem and our attempts to develop an effective and appropriate public response to it. Because of the social meanings of AIDS, these issues are restricted to the logic of effective public health planning.

## A CHALLENGE TO INDIVIDUAL LIBERTY

The development of public health policies on AIDS is complicated enormously by its multiply stigmatized character. The public identification of people infected with the AIDS virus that would be required under many proposed screening programs would alienate individuals from their communities and livelihoods just as effectively as frank policies of isolation or quarantine. Such policies could be seen as unjustifiable infringements on individual freedom of action and association. AIDS, in other words, is also a civil liberties problem. Thus, the chapters in Part Three all examine the potential social dangers of discriminatory and coercive disease control policies. In their chapters, Carol Tauer and Paul Carrick chart the terrain of policy interventions and explore the philosophical constructs that underlie policy options. The other authors in Part Three scrutinize particular policies: Jacqueline Glover and Edward Starkeson discuss the screening of health care professionals, Timothy Murphy looks at quarantines, Andrew Moss analyses the San Francisco decision to close gay bathhouses, and John Moskop explores a range of public screening campaigns.

The authors in Part Three all emphasize that assessments of the scien-

tific effectiveness of restrictive public health measures are inevitably influenced by the stigmatized nature of the illness. Many of the policies
these authors discuss as possibilities are already being implemented in
some communities in the United States. As a result, the authors' philosophical analyses have gained a particularly vivid timeliness and underscore the very practical value of attempting to untangle the many meanings of AIDS.

## ACKNOWLEDGMENTS

The chapters in this volume originated as contributions to the 1986
Spring National Meeting of the Society for Health and Human Values,
"AIDS and the Medical Humanities," held in San Francisco. The conference was cohosted by the Division of Medical Ethics and the Department
of History of Health Sciences at the University of California at San Francisco. The chapters were revised and edited for this volume. We grateful-
ly acknowledge financial support for the conference from the Walter and
Elise Haas Foundation and from the California Council for the Humanities, a state affiliate of the National Endowment for the Humanities. The
findings, conclusions, and opinions presented here do not necessarily
represent the views of the Haas Foundation, the California Council for
the Humanities, or the National Endowment for the Humanities.

We are indebted to many individuals within this framework of financial and institutional support: George Degnon and Carol O'Neil at the
Society for Health and Human Values, Albert Jonsen and Guenter Risse
at the University of California, and Caitlin Croughan at the California
Council for the Humanities. We would also like to thank Stephen Arkin
for assisting with the essential but unrewarding details of editorial work
and Rose Martinez, whose word processing skills were, in the end, the
key to the volume's realization.

## NOTES

1. We are indebted to Albert Jonsen for this metaphor, which he used in his
introduction to the conference for which the chapters in this volume were
written.

2. P. Conrad, The social meanings of AIDS. *Social Policy* 17 (1986):51–56.

# I  Interpreting Our Knowledge of AIDS

# 1 NAMING THE AIDS VIRUS
## Harold E. Varmus

Between April 1983 and August 1984, three research groups in three locales 3,000 miles apart reported the isolation of viruses advanced as candidates for the causative agent of the acquired immunodeficiency syndrome (AIDS).[1] Although these viruses were called different names by each of the laboratories that reported them, the many isolates now appear to form a very closely related virus group within the much larger and well-studied class known as retroviruses.[2] By the end of 1984, it was apparent that both the scientific community and the public would be better served by a single name for the causative agent of AIDS, but it was much less clear what that name should be or what criteria should be applied to decide on it.

Beginning in March 1985, I chaired a committee composed of 13 retrovirologists from four countries, which was to attempt to find a single acceptable name for this important new group of human retroviruses. This duty of serving as chair fell to me because I head a standing subcommittee, known as the Retrovirus Study Group, which is empowered to rule on matters of retroviral nomenclature and classification under the aegis of a larger group known as the International Committee on the Taxonomy of Viruses. We were summoned to action on this occasion by calls and letters from virologists close to and distant from the experimental activity, asking that some neutral group offer a solution to what had become an intractably confusing and at times overtly contentious issue.

The normal workings of our study group are sporadic, often pedantic, and of little concern to the general public, though useful to those who

3

must work with and talk about viruses. In the case of the AIDS virus, however, our activities have attracted extraordinary attention and curiosity.

Why has there been so much interest in the resolution of a problem that would appear to have no immediate relevance to the serious issues in the AIDS crisis—controlling the spread of this virus and treating its victims? Some perceive, wrongly in my view, that our final recommendation will form a verdict upon contested issues of priority of discovery, issues that could influence patent rights, the awarding of major prizes, patriotic sentiments, and financial gain. Others have seen our deliberations as a battle between Robert Gallo and Luc Montagnier, both members of the committee and leaders of the two most highly publicized groups to isolate AIDS retroviruses. This is certainly an oversimplified view of the proceedings. For many who follow the AIDS problem closely as experimental scientists, health care workers, or public-spirited citizens, the issue may simply be one of having a single, convenient, and generally accepted name for the virus that causes the disease. And for an appreciable number of scientists, the task has a higher purpose, eloquently expressed by Stephen Jay Gould: " . . . taxonomies are not neutral hatracks for the pristine facts of nature. They are theories that create and reflect the deep structure of science and human culture. A taxonomy is not just a ploy for convenient arrangement, but a hypothetical statement about the nature of things."

In fact, the issue before us has not been taxonomy per se, but nomenclature; we have attempted to settle upon what is usually called the common or species name for a virus or collection of very similar viruses. Since such names are in daily use by the working virologist, much ink and some blood have been spilled over them. The forces that influence decisions about them are as various as the forces that influence the naming of a baby, a book, a bridge, or a city.

Scientific principles, political realities, aesthetics, convention, and justice must all be served in the process of finding the species name for a virus. Many questions had to be considered for each suggestion: Is the proposed name consistent with scientific facts and with the tentative classification of the virus? Is there anything objectionable about the name that would prevent its being used? Have those credited with discovery been accorded their right to contribute to the process of naming? Does the name distinguish the virus from those it does not resemble? Is the name readily remembered? Is the name likely to create confusion in the future if and when other viruses are isolated? Does the name conform to existing conventions for naming viruses of this general type?

Before discussing specific names proposed for the AIDS virus, I must briefly introduce a debate that has been raging among namers of viruses for the past few years. The definition of an animal species is based upon the ability to mate productively; membership in a species is granted to those animals that can interbreed with other members. Since viruses do not have sex in the conventional sense, the grouping of viruses that are so closely related as to be accorded a common name has often been based upon any conveniently measured biological or biochemical property, such as virus shape, or immune reactivity, or the presence of a certain enzyme in the virus particle.

With the application of new genetic and molecular techniques to the study of viruses, however, it has become possible to define virus groups in a fashion analogous to that used for animals; that is, in a way that is likely to come closer to establishing true evolutionary relationships among viruses.[3] In this new view, it is possible to assess which viruses are so closely related genetically that they could exchange genes without loss of viability, in the manner of animals that can generate viable offspring by the intermingling of their genes. Such viruses properly constitute a species and can usually be clearly distinguished from those that are genetically disparate, regardless of other similarities.

In the context of the AIDS viruses, for example, it was apparent by the time our deliberations began that the available isolates were sufficiently closely related to be considered members of the same virus species. The questions, in large part, were whether and how they should be distinguished from human retroviruses that appeared to belong to other species by genetic criteria.

What names did we have to consider? Several names were already in use. Most prominent among these were lymphadenopathy virus (LAV), human T-cell lymphotropic virus-III (HTLV-III), AIDS-associated retrovirus (ARV), two hybrid names (HTLV-III/LAV and LAV/HTLV-III), and a name often used by the press (the AIDS virus). In short order, many more names, about 50 counting all permutations, were suggested by committee members, consultants, and other correspondents.

How could we decide among these many candidates? When confronted by confusion, it is sometimes useful to consider what had worked well in the past. Retroviruses form a large group of agents united by a distinctive property: They carry their genes in the form of ribonucleic acid (RNA) and convert the genes to deoxyribonucleic acid (DNA) after infection, reversing the usual flow of information in nature from DNA to RNA. Despite this unifying feature, retroviruses are also manifestly diverse: They are found in many different animal hosts, cause several different types of disease, and frequently appear to be only marginally related when the substance of their genes is carefully examined.[4] This complexity has generated a need to group isolates in a rational manner that emphasizes biological boundaries.

Traditional retroviral nomenclature has worked well in this regard. The convention has been to name viruses according to the host species of

origin and the prominent pathology associated with the prototypic isolate of a single type; two examples of such names are feline leukemia
virus and mouse mammary tumor virus. Individual isolates belonging to
a single species are further distinguished by prefixes or suffixes [num-
bers, letters, or (in earlier times) names of discoverers], as in Rauscher
murine leukemia virus or human T-cell leukemia virus-2.

Many of us have favored staying close to these traditional rules, but
there were obviously other considerations as well. In particular, the
rights of discoverers had to be respected, but it was clear from the outset
that we could not reach a consensus about eminent domain. It thus
seemed prudent to set as an objective the best possible name, to include
all claimants in the proceedings, and to hope that all parties would find
some solution acceptable.

If we were to adopt a traditional name for the AIDS retrovirus, we
needed to consider a particularly troubling issue: whether names that
included the term AIDS, such as human AIDS virus or human AIDS-
lymphadenopathy virus, were likely to be psychologically damaging in
the clinic, in view of the lethality of the disease and the social stigmas
attached to the prevalent routes of virus transmission. To explore this
issue, we asked over 50 clinicians who had worked with AIDS patients
for their opinions. The large number who responded showed genuine
and intelligent interest in the choice of names, but they were almost
exactly divided over the issue of whether to exclude "AIDS" from the
name. Some took the position that patients would soon be as fearful
about any term that denoted the agent of AIDS as about a term that was
explicit, a phenomenon our committee referred to as "the evanescence of
euphemism." Others felt strongly that it would be easier to explain the
difference between infection by the virus and the disease itself subsequently induced in a minority of infected people if the virus had a name
with less pejorative potential.

There was general agreement among our membership that the latter
view should prevail, if only because strict adherence to simplicity and
convention was not important enough to outweigh the misfortune of
even a rare patient's suffering needlessly from the report of an antibody
test. Moreover, it was possible to consider use of terms that denote the
principal pathological consequences of infection—for example, "immunodeficiency" or "immunosuppression"—thereby avoiding the name
of the disease, yet conforming to standard nomenclature.

The many names suggested for the AIDS virus raised other taxonomic
possibilities. Some encouraged the use of host cell affinity (tropism) as a
basis for the name, a view already in wide circulation through the use of
the term "human T-cell lymphotropic virus" and endorsed by other suggestions, such as "human T4 virus," which names the cellular receptor
that determines whether the virus can enter a cell. (This approach is

discussed more fully below.) Another possibility was raised by experimental evidence linking the AIDS virus with a handful of animal retroviruses that produce disease slowly and are hence known as lentiviruses, one of the three large subgroups of retroviruses.[5] However, enthusiasm for "human lentivirus-1" was dampened by the still weakly defined characteristics of this class and by the inappropriateness of using as a species name a name normally applied to a collection of diverse virus species. Others suggested defusing the political, clinical, and genetic issues through the use of a sequential numbering system, in which the AIDS virus could become "human retrovirus-3." However, colorless names of this type can be difficult to connect with the right virus, especially when the list becomes lengthy: The approach does not respect the genetic basis of virus speciation, since human retroviruses from different species would have names that differ only by number, and attempts to impose similar systems upon other virus groups, such as human herpesviruses, have not always been successful.

From a pragmatic perspective, we had to consider the already widespread use of the term human T-cell lymphotropic virus-III (HTLV-III) and to ask whether it was too firmly entrenched to be displaced by a new name. This tactical question, however, was accompanied by the theoretical issue of how modern virologists view the world and how they recreate it for their students through the choice of names, because the term HTLV-III presents a direct challenge to the genetic basis of virus speciation.

Proponents of HTLV-III wished to group it with HTLV-I and HTLV-II—viruses originally called human T-cell leukemia viruses, but proposed to be renamed as T-cell lymphotropic viruses—on the basis of a long list of common features.[6] However, the most prominent of these similarities appear superficial and deceptive when closely examined. Thus, though both virus types have strong predilections for infecting the T4 subset of thymus-derived lymphocytes, the mechanisms determining that preference are fundamentally different for the leukemia viruses and the AIDS virus. In the first place, the two groups of viruses use different host cell receptors to gain entry into the lymphocytes; as a consequence, they also differ with regard to other cell types they can infect. Second, though the leukemia and AIDS viruses are pathogenic for humans, they cause dramatically different types of pathology that result, on the one hand, from the inappropriate proliferation of infected cells (leukemia) and, on the other, from toxicity and the death of infected cells (AIDS). Third, despite several similarities in the sizes of the proteins found in leukemia and AIDS virus particles, the sequences of the building blocks (amino acids) of these proteins are now known to be as different as the sequences for any two ostensibly unrelated retroviruses. Finally, though both types of viruses exhibit relatively unusual mechanisms for improving the efficiency with which they produce the proteins encoded by their genes, on close inspection the mechanisms appear to be largely unrelated.[7]

The explanation of these fundamental differences is immediately apparent when the viral chromosomes (known as genomes) are compared.[8] Though the genomes of the AIDS and leukemia viruses share features that are common to all retroviruses—units at the ends to govern gene expression and a basic layout of genes for the proteins found in virus particles—wherever they can differ, they do. Most obviously, the order of the components of the genome differs, so that the sequence of nucleotides is no more similar for these two groups than for any two members of the diverse family of retroviruses. But important subtleties are also evident: The manner in which the major genes are juxtaposed assigns the viruses to different classes, and the position and nature of other genes are entirely unrelated.

If an evolutionary tree is established for retroviruses by comparing the order of amino acids in the protein most characteristic of retroviruses, that is, reverse transcriptase, the enzyme that converts RNA to DNA, it is apparent that the AIDS virus is most closely related to the sheep lentivirus, called visna, whereas the human T-cell leukemia viruses are in another limb of the tree, more closely related to other cancer-causing viruses, such as leukemia and sarcoma viruses of various animals, particularly the bovine leukemia virus.[9] To those who believe in the application of genetic principles to virus nomenclature, it is apparent that a superficial resemblance in host cell tropism should not be used to impose a species designation upon viruses that are highly divergent according to more rigorous criteria.

Through a series of memoranda and polls that sought a consensus on these issues, exchanging views almost exclusively by telephone or mail, we narrowed the choices to a few, then identified a name approved by a resounding majority but not by acclamation. (That name and the letter officially proposing it to the scientific community are presented in the Postscript at the end of this chapter.) The issue that remains is a practical one: Can we bring this name into common use? Or will we simply have added an academic suggestion, albeit one enshrined in the official logs of an international agency, to the list of names already in use?

Colleagues sometimes ask why we should care about this issue, with convictions that go beyond the usual manifestations of good scientific citizenship. During our deliberations, at least two components of our commitment have emerged. As proponents of the disciplines of virology and genetics, we want them to operate in a way that seems to us and to students we train to be scientifically sound. Moreover, we would like the public view of our science to be one that acknowledges the reality of disagreement, but one that also admires the willingness of intellectual combatants to compromise in order to advance our shared purpose. A prolonged battle over the issue of a name for the AIDS virus is more than trivial because the battle may come—some might say it has come—to symbolize certain excesses of character for which scientists are often criticized. This seems particularly unfortunate in view of the truly extraordinary accomplishments that have been made in a very short time by the laboratories involved in the debate. A generally accepted recommendation for a name for this virus could help restore to the public whatever faith has been lost through this issue during the confusion of the past two years.

## POSTSCRIPT

During the first week of May 1986, the following letter from our subcommittee appeared in the journals *Nature* and *Science*. Two members of our group, Myron Essex and Robert Gallo, declined to sign the agreement.

To the Editor:

The undersigned are members of a subcommittee empowered by the International Committee on the Taxonomy of Viruses to propose an appropriate name for the retrovirus isolates recently implicated as the causative agents of the acquired immune deficiency syndrome (AIDS). Adoption of an internationally-acceptable name for this group of viruses has become an important issue because of the widespread interest in AIDS and its origins and because of the names currently in use. Thus the several isolates of what are now evidently closely related members of the same virus group have been called lymphadenopathy associated virus (LAV), human T-cell lymphotropic virus type III (HTLV-III), immunodeficiency associated virus (IDAV), and AIDS-associated retrovirus (ARV). At present, two compound names (HTLV-III/LAV and LAV/HTLV-III) are also used in scientific publications, and the colloquial name, the AIDS virus, is often used by the press.

We are writing to propose that the AIDS retroviruses be officially designated as the human immunodeficiency viruses, to be known in abbreviated form as HIV.

We have considered several issues that bear upon this proposal. (i) The name conforms to common nomenclature for retroviruses, beginning with the host species ("human"), ending with "virus," and containing a word that denotes a major (though not the only) pathogenetic property of the prototypic members of the group ("immunodeficiency"). ("Feline leukemia virus" and "mouse mammary tumor virus" are two well-known examples of such names for retrovirus species.) (ii) Though the name clearly connects the viruses to the disease with which the virus group is associated, it does not incorporate the term "AIDS," which many clinicians urged us to avoid. (iii) The name is readily distinguished from all existing names for this group of viruses and has been chosen without regard to priority of discovery. (iv) The name is sufficiently distinct from the names of other retroviruses to imply an independent virus species, a group of isolates that can presumably exchange genetic information readily with each other but not with members of other known retrovirus species. These other species include the human T-cell leukemia viruses (e.g., HTLV-1 and -2), which will continue to be named according to a convention adopted by several leading investigators in September, 1983. (Though roman numerals are often used to indicate the type of HTLV, arabic numbers were originally prescribed in the agreement and are thus used here.) (v) Retroviruses isolated from subhuman primates and found to be genetically related and biologically similar to HIV's should be designated as immunodeficiency viruses of the appropriate host species [e.g., simian immunodeficiency virus (SIV) or African green monkey immunodeficiency virus (AGMIV)]. (vi) Because HIV isolates are numerous and display considerable genetic heterogeneity, particularly in the *env* gene, it will be necessary for each laboratory to assign subspecies designations to [its] isolates. We recommend that each laboratory adopt a code with geographically informative letters and sequential numbers to identify their isolates (e.g., the 42nd isolate at the University of Chicago could be described as HIV [CHI-42]). Initially, the existing, well-characterized isolates, such as LAV-1, HTLV-IIIB, or ARV-2, should be identified as such in publications to ease the transition to a unified nomenclature. (vii) Any future isolates of human retroviruses with clear but limited relationship to isolates of HIV (e.g., more than 20 percent but less than 50 percent nucleic acid sequence identity) should not be called HIV unless there are compelling biological and structural similarities to existing members of the group.

We hope that this proposal will be adopted rapidly by the research community working with the viruses.

John Coffin
Tufts University, Medford, MA

Ashley Haase
University of Minnesota, Minneapolis, MN

Jay A. Levy
University of California, San Francisco, CA

Luc Montagnier
Pasteur Institute, Paris, France

Stephen Oroszlan
Frederick Cancer Research Center, Frederick, MD

Natalie Teich
Imperial Cancer Research Fund, London, England

Howard Temin
University of Wisconsin, Madison, WI

Kumao Toyoshima
University of Tokyo, Tokyo, Japan

Harold Varmus, Chairman
University of California, San Francisco, CA

Peter Vogt
University of Southern California, Los Angeles, CA

Robin Weiss
Institute of Cancer Research, Chester Beatty Laboratories, London, England

Reprinted by permission from *Nature*, Vol. 321, p. 10, Copyright © 1986 Macmillan Magazines Limited; and *Science*, Vol. 232, pp. 697–98, Copyright © 1986 by the AAAS.

## NOTES

1. F. Barre-Sinoussi, et al., Isolation of T-lymphotropic retrovirus from a patient at risk for acquired immune deficiency syndrome (AIDS). *Science* 220 (1983):868–70; R. C. Gallo, et al., Human T-lymphotropic retrovirus, HTLV-III, isolated from AIDS patients and donors at risk for AIDS. *Science* 224 (1984):500–503; J. A. Levy, et al., Isolation of lymphocytopathic retroviruses from San Francisco patients with AIDS. *Science* 225 (1984):840–42.

2. R. Weiss. Human T-cell retroviruses. In *RNA Tumor Viruses, Molecular Biology of Tumor Viruses*. 2nd ed. Vol. 2. Ed. R. Weiss, et al. Cold Spring Harbor, NY: Cold Spring Harbor Laboratory, 1985, pp. 405–85.

3. D. W. Kingsbury. Species classification problems in virus taxonomy. *Intervirology* 24 (1985):62–70.

4. Kingsbury, Species classification problems.

5. N. Teich. Taxonomy of retroviruses. In *RNA Tumor Viruses, Molecular Biology of Tumor Viruses*. 2nd ed. Vol. 1. Ed. R. Weiss, et al. Cold Spring Harbor, NY: Cold Spring Harbor Laboratory, 1985, pp. 25–27.

6. S. Wain-Hobson, M. Alizon, and L. Montagnier. Relationship of AIDS to other retroviruses. *Nature* 313 (1985):743.

7. F. Wong-Staal and R. C. Gallo. Human T-lymphotropic retroviruses. *Nature* 317 (1985):395–403.

8. C. A. Rosen, et al., Post-transcriptional regulation accounts for the trans-activation of the human T-lymphotropic virus type III. *Nature* 319 (1986):555–59.

9. Teich, Taxonomy of retroviruses.

# 2  CAUSAL EXPLANATIONS OF AIDS
*Jana L. Armstrong*

> Knowledge is the object of our inquiry, and men do not think they
> know a thing till they have grasped the "why" of it (which is to grasp
> its primary cause).
>
> —Aristotle, *Physics*

In February 1985, a congressional report announced that "the basic
cause of acquired immunodeficiency syndrome (AIDS) is almost certainly a newly discovered virus, human T-cell lymphotropic virus, type III,
or HTLV-III."[1] What does it mean to call this thing that we now name the
HIV virus the *basic* cause of AIDS? The word "cause" is embedded in the
language of public policy, the language of cell biology, the language of
epidemiology. But the word does not mean the same thing in every
instance of its use. The word "cause" seems to penetrate the discourse of
these fields somewhat in the manner in which a virus is thought to
penetrate human bodies—producing different results in each one and
yet somehow still displaying the same essence.

To understand how we think about AIDS, it is useful to look at the way
we organize our knowledge about causation in medicine. To identify a
causal relationship is to respond to the question why? in a particular
way. An examination of causal explanations can thus yield important
information about the aims of the disciplines that employ them. A careful examination of biomedical discourse about AIDS can reveal whether
we speak of AIDS the way we do by absolute necessity (that is, because
of an imperative of language), or whether a certain economy (use of

familiar concepts and terms) and a certain strategy (aims in thus employing these concepts and terms) are at work.

The discovery of the AIDS virus was credited to the joint efforts of researchers who published a collection of four articles concerning the identification of the virus and its association with AIDS in *Science*, in May 1984.[2] In their initial report they "proposed that AIDS may be caused by a virus from the [HTLV] family"[3] and in another article in the same issue they "suggest that HTLV-III is the primary cause of AIDS."[4] A later report in *Science* cites the previous articles but states with more certitude: "Human T-cell lymphotropic virus (HTLV-III/LAV)[5] is the etiologic agent of the acquired immunodeficiency syndrome (AIDS)."[6] "Etiologic agent" is defined as "the cause of a disease or disorder as determined by medical diagnosis."[7] This announcement has had interesting effects on the discourse about AIDS. For example, it would seem like the discovery that AIDS is caused by a virus would effectively dispose of any notion that AIDS is caused by homosexual men. Yet this has not been the case. Reports from biological researchers that they have found the "basic" or "primary" cause of AIDS has done little to dispel previously conceived ideas about what does, or does not, cause AIDS. This is because we do not use "cause" as a univocal term.

When researchers refer to the AIDS virus as the *primary* cause of the disease, this constitutes more than a rhetorical flourish. It implies a particular, historically well-determined epistemological basis.

In order to understand the role of cause in the medical sciences, we must consider its beginnings in Western philosophy. Aristotle set forth a fourfold notion of causation in the *Physics*.[8] By looking at the way the term "cause" is used by those investigating AIDS (specifically those concerned with immunological cell biology and epidemiology) through the lens of Aristotle's categories of causation, we can begin to understand why there can be no single, basic, or primary cause of AIDS.

Aristotle's theory of causation clarifies causes into four types: material cause, formal cause, final cause, and efficient cause. Whether a cause is necessary or incidental or whether it is due to human intelligence or to nature, these four categories exhaust the formal dimensions of causation. Today in the natural sciences the type (or types) of cause invoked varies according to the mode of investigation, but it is usually possible to identify one or more of Aristotle's categories at work.

## MATERIAL CAUSE

Aristotle defined material cause as "that out of which a thing comes to be and which persists, . . . e.g. the bronze of the statue, the silver of the bowl. . . ."[9] In this sense, the biochemical analysis of the AIDS virus investigates cause at a molecular level. Quantitative analysis of the molecular weights of antigenic proteins, for example, is thought to reveal the nature of the virus's biological substances. Thus, the reactivities of the antibodies in the sera of AIDS patients are tested in order to estimate the molecular weights of the antigenic protein with which they react.[10] When this analysis is conducted on serum antibodies collected from AIDS patients, persons at "increased risk" of contracting AIDS, and "normal" controls, characteristic patterns of protein binding are observed. It was such a pattern that was used to design the ELISA, or enzyme-linked immunosorbent assay, test. This test indicates whether the antibodies in an individual's blood bind to proteins in a fashion similar or dissimilar (within accepted ranges) to that of antibodies in blood exposed to the AIDS virus.

But the biochemical description of HIV (human immunodeficiency virus) alone does not produce a causal explanation. Biochemistry is distinct from physicochemistry in that the former is concerned with living things—explanations are not proffered without some reference to biological organisms. The detection and isolation of the AIDS virus is made possible by growing cell cultures that not only can be subjected to assay tests but can be scrutinized under the electron microscope. In this way the virus makes an "appearance" and Aristotle's second notion of cause, formal cause, is invoked.

## FORMAL CAUSE

Aristotle defines formal cause as "the form or the archetype, i.e. the statement of the essence. . . . "[11] Form defines the common attributes of a species, the qualities that are replicated in each individual. Although it is somewhat problematic to consider a virus as a living organism,[12] the description of the AIDS virus nonetheless conforms to Aristotle's category of formal cause. Recall the two-step process that was involved in defining the essential properties of HTLV-III. First there was the analytic procedure of *assimilation*—a virus of the HTLV family was implicated by analogy with the previously determined properties of HTLV viruses. Seven such properties were identified in the description of HTLV-III, including the observation that "another retrovirus, feline leukemia virus, causes immune deficiency in cats," that "retroviruses of the HTLV family are T-cell tropic," and that HTLV-family viruses "may be transmitted by intimate contact and blood products."[13]

The next step consisted of *differentiation*: It had to be shown that HTLV-III was different from the other members of the HTLV family. The "somewhat different" morphology of HTLV-III under the electron microscope and "some differences found in the protein patterns of purified virus preparations"[14] were suggested as a basis for this distinction. As an example of a difference in protein patterns, the low level of antibody reaction in the sera of AIDS patients to gp61, a glycoprotein that occurs in a cell line producing HTLV-I virus, was cited. Thus, differences in HTLV viruses were identified both quantitatively (through antibody titers and the analysis of molecular weights of antigens) and visually (using the electron microscope to examine HTLV-III cell staining or by examining immunoblot or immunosorbent assays). On the one hand, we have a linguistic operation; assimilation and differentiation are both processes necessary to the production of a definition. On the other hand, we have laboratory procedures which, while guided by rules, are interpretive and hence dependent upon human sensibilities.

In a more recent article, researchers continue the search for purified forms.[15] The two immunogenic proteins p66 and p51, acting in a dependent fashion, are said to characterize the reverse transcriptase (the enzyme that characterizes retroviruses) of HTLV-III. In other words, antibodies in the blood sera of 80 percent of HTLV-III antibody-positive individuals in a random sample recognized, or reacted with, these two proteins, which had been extracted in "purified" form.[16] What this notion of "purified" form implies is that the presence or absence of the identical virus (or its antibodies, in the case of the ELISA test) can be determined in blood sample after blood sample.

But we really have not said much about cause by identifying the material substances involved and the pure forms they assume. For one thing, the presence of the AIDS virus in blood sera has *not* been shown by researchers to be either a necessary or sufficient condition for contracting the disease AIDS. In other words, persons who test positive for antibodies to the AIDS virus do not have AIDS, and persons who have AIDS do not always test positive for antibodies. If the presence of the virus is not coextensive with AIDS, then by virtue of what rigorous logic or natural law do we assign the term "basic" or "primary cause" to the viral agent?

## FINAL CAUSE

The AIDS virus cannot be thought of as *the* cause of AIDS unless the virus is assigned a purpose in an ordered biological universe. This brings us to the third form of causation—final, or teleological, cause. Aristotle defined final cause as the end, or "that for the sake of which" a thing is done.[17] By assigning the role of pathogen to the virus, we can construct a narrative about its reason for being. For example, a researcher might talk about the *function* of the virus in the destruction of a patient's immune system. The purposeful role of the virus as the agent causing AIDS is axiomatic—not a fact inevitably arising from consideration of the evidence. Statistical associations should not be confused with causal explanations; neither should a quantitative analogy be taken for a necessary and sufficient condition, particularly when the research in question affirms that it is not.

Mistaking the hypothetical for the absolute is not an inconsequential error. It can provide scientific legitimation for policies that serve to distinguish between individuals in terms of, for example, their ability to transmit the disease we call AIDS. This ability to "fractionate" (to use a term employed by researchers)[18] a society on the basis of a scientific test becomes crucial when we consider Aristotle's fourth and last notion of cause: efficient cause.

## EFFICIENT CAUSE

Aristotle defines efficient cause as "the primary source of change or coming to rest; e.g. the man who gave advice is a cause, the father is the cause of the child, and generally what makes of what is made and what causes change of what is changed."[19] In this way, says Aristotle, "a man" could be said to be the cause of a thing. Following this line of thinking, we perceive that the AIDS virus does not produce change independently, does not single-handedly introduce chaotic disease into a naturally hermetic, ordered world of immunity. As a disease transmissible through intimate contact and blood products, AIDS needs an *efficient cause*, a "transmitter of what is transmitted." To fully know its cause, we would have to know what efficient agent brings about the mingling of blood products and/or semen.

Here epidemiologists take over the question of cause when they identify "high-risk groups." Officials of the Centers for Disease Control linked homosexuality, intravenous drug use, and the transmission of the AIDS virus in a causal argument when they stated: "The initial occurrence of the syndrome among homosexual men and intravenous drug users suggested a transmissible agent as the cause."[20] But what might public health officials *mean* when they say that homosexuals, hemophiliacs, Haitians, or heroin addicts (as opposed to say, "San Franciscans") are at increased risk of contracting AIDS? They imply that being homosexual can be the *efficient cause* of an individual's disease. They are selecting those characteristics of individuals that the epidemiologist thinks (according to some prior logic) make them suspect of being efficient transmitters, or conversely, victims, of disease.

The underlying argument is as follows: It is that man's being homosexual which made of him a transmitter (or a victim) of AIDS. We have yet to discover, however, what *specifically* makes a homosexual a likely carrier of AIDS. In fact, the analytic usefulness of the category of homosexual becomes questionable when you consider that the criteria used to determine the boundaries of what is or is not homosexuality vary and are usually not made explicit. This determination is sometimes made on the basis of self-reported sexual preference (a subjective statement) or on the basis that the person had sexual relations with someone of the same sex (a description of actual behavior). In order for this epidemiology of homosexuality to sustain credibility, it would have to account for these discrepancies. A more precise determination of what constitutes homosexuality in rigorous scientific terms would have to be made. The epidemiologist would have to undertake the task of defining homosexuals in terms of essential attributes—no easy feat. And this alone would not suffice. The constitution of homosexuality as a proper object of scientific study requires that these attributes be discoverable and that they uniquely define homosexuals.

But the characterization of AIDS as a homosexual disease had proceeded without the benefit of a scientific definition of homosexuality. Amidst such ambiguity, epidemiologic reporting has led to the confusion of categories—for example, the practice of anal intercourse with homosexuality, or homosexuality with promiscuity. Again, these are not inconsequential confusions. Implying that a person's sexual preference or Haitian nationality can be the *efficient cause* of disease affords scientific legitimacy to policies that limit the scope of action of such persons "in the interest of public health," for example, by quarantine, expulsion from the army, or denial of access to public places, employment, and housing. In so doing we mask social or psychological statements by labeling them as empirical. We take statistical correlations and confuse them with necessary or sufficient conditions for disease. And as a consequence, we lend implicit support to teleological statements such as "homosexuality is the cause of AIDS."

But is there not a sense in which the efficient cause of a thing, the "maker of what is made," is the one who discloses the cause of a thing in both its form and its matter, assigns it a teleological purpose, and gives it a name? Before we had a name for the AIDS virus, could define its chemical properties, and could see the reflected image of its constituent parts under the electron microscope, we could not talk about viral infection. We could only talk about an unusual number of deaths due to opportunistic infection or Kaposi's sarcoma in previously healthy individuals, and relate these deaths to the selected qualities or self-avowed behaviors of AIDS victims. Now, in light of basic viral research, we seem to have a much more concrete grasp of the cause of AIDS. And this, of course, is due to the work of physicians who report AIDS cases; public health officials who process this data; biochemists, virologists, and immunologists who report their research; politicians who affirm or repudiate their findings; the journalistic media that disseminate this information; and, of course, those of us who choose to study and discuss this information. These are the individuals who consider, gather together, and bring into view the nature or essence of the cause of AIDS. And there is a legitimate sense in which "the maker of the thing made" is the agent who carries out this process of revealing.

## CONCLUSION

The preceding suggests that in speaking or writing about the AIDS virus as being the *cause* of AIDS, we may be attaching a surplus of meaning to the object of our investigation. This surplus of meaning results when a virus is identified as being causally, rather than merely statistically, linked with AIDS. Conversely, to attempt to speak about the AIDS virus without any reference to causation might distort the meaning of the name HTLV-III (or HIV). Viruses are essentially and ontologically defined as infectious, that is, capable of *causing* infection. If the role of a virus as causal agent is cast into question, the force of signification attached to the term HTLV-III (or HIV) is seriously undermined.

The role of cause in the discourse of medicine and biological science requires further attention. To proceed as if empirical truth could be independent of language is to simply eliminate the role of interpretation in scientific investigation. But as long as the discourse about AIDS continues to concern causation, the role of interpretation will be crucial. This is because cause is precisely that "thing" to which we will never have purely empirical access.

Auguste Comte's *Cours de philosophie positive* describes the goal of positivistic (or natural) philosophy:

We see, from the preceding, that the fundamental character of positive philosophy is to consider phenomena as subject to natural, invariable laws, of which the precise discovery and reduction to the least number possible are the goal of all of our efforts, considering as absolutely inaccessible and empty of sense for us the investigation of what are called *causes*, whether first or final.[21]

The reason given for excluding causes from the field of positivistic investigation is that they are *inaccessible*. Cause somehow lies outside the realm of experience. The positivistic, empirical sciences have been modified since *Cours de philosophie positive* was published, but they have not explicitly reappropriated the investigation of causes that Comte categorically rejected. Empirical studies aim at describing relationships between things, not at determining the *nature* of these relationships. In other words, an event may be said to be the antecedent of another event, and these events may occur in succession with a certain frequency. But the determination that the one is the cause of the other would not, according to the positivistic position, be a matter of scientific import.

If cause were taken as a topic outside the domain of scientific inquiry, then what would we make of the term when it is employed in medical literature? If cause can never be subjected directly to experience, how then can cause be investigated?

Cause is, from the outset, inscribed in a gesture of interpretation. It is in a piecemeal and fragmentary way that we know the cause of AIDS, because we know the cause in a discursive way. It may be suggested that piecemeal and fragmentary knowledge about AIDS is better than no knowledge at all—but this type of judgment is not scientific. It is moral and political.

Aristotle defined the conditions for a scientific investigation of cause:

We suppose ourselves to possess unqualified scientific knowledge of a thing, as opposed to knowing it in the accidental way in which the sophist knows, when we think that we know the cause on which the fact depends, as the cause of that fact and no other, and, further, that the fact could not be other than it is.[22]

That last requirement is indeed a strict one. It is so strict, in fact, that it raises the question of whether or not medicine and the biological disciplines can *scientifically* speak of cause and at the same time be said to be speaking scientifically? If they cannot, this will inform our reading of medicine and the biological sciences in general, and our interpretation of AIDS in particular.

## NOTES

[Editors' note: In this chapter the name of the viral agent has not been changed to HIV because the author refers to a specific time period before HIV became the accepted nomenclature.]

1. Office of Technology Assessment, Congress of the United States. *A Technical Memorandum: Review of the Public Health Services' Response to AIDS*. Washington, D.C.: U.S. Government Printing Office, February 1985.

2. M. Popovic et al. Detection, isolation, and continuous production of cytopathic retroviruses (HTLV-III) from patients with AIDS and pre-AIDS. *Science* 224 (1984):497–500; R. C. Gallo et al. Frequent detection and isolation of cytopathic retroviruses (HTLV-III) from patients with AIDS and at risk for AIDS. *Science* 224 (1984):500–3; J. Schupbach et al. Serological analysis of a subgroup of human T-lymphotropic retroviruses (HTLV-III) associated with AIDS. *Science* 224 (1984): 503–5; M. G. Sarngadharan et al. Antibodies reactive with human T-lymphotropic retroviruses (HTLV-III) in serum of patients with AIDS. *Science* 224 (1984): 506–8.

3. Popovic et al., Detection, 497.

4. Sarngadharan et al., Antibodies, 508.

5. The change in name from HTLV-III to HTLV-III/LAV indicates that Gallo and his coauthors acknowledge that the virus called LAV by French researchers at the Pasteur Institute is substantially identical to HTLV-III.

6. F. D. Veronese, T. D. Copeland, R. R. DeVico, et al. Characterization of

highly immunogenic p66/p51 as the reverse transcriptase of HTLV-III/LAV. *Science* 231 (1986):1289–91.

7. *American Heritage Dictionary of the English Language*. New York: Houghton Mifflin, 1973.

8. R. McKeon. *Introduction to Aristotle*, 2nd ed., revised and enlarged. Chicago: University of Chicago Press, 1973.

9. Ibid., 128.

10. Veronese et al., Characterization, 1290.

11. McKeon, *Introduction to Aristotle*, 128.

12. The following definition of virus (taken from *Dorland's Illustrated Medical Dictionary*, Philadelphia: W. B. Saunders, 1981) suggests that viruses are *not* living organisms in only *like* living organisms:

One of a group of minute infectious agents, with certain exceptions (e.g. pox viruses) not resolved in the light microscope, and characterized by a lack of independent metabolism and by the ability to replicate only within living host cells. Like living organisms, they are able to reproduce with genetic continuity and the possibility of mutation. . . .

13. Popovic et al., Detection, 497.

14. Ibid., 505.

15. Veronese et al., Characterization, 1290.

16. Ibid., 1289–90.

17. McKeon, *Introduction to Aristotle*, 128.

18. Veronese et al., Characterization, 1289–90.

19. McKeon, *Introduction to Aristotle*, 128.

20. J. W. Curran et al. The epidemiology of AIDS: Current status and future prospects. *Science* 229 (1984):1352–57.

21. A. Comte. *Cours de philosophie positive*. 2nd ed. First Lesson. Paris: J. B. Bailliere et Fils, Librairie de l'Academie Imperiale de Médecine, 1864, p. 16 (author's translation).

22. McKeon, *Introduction to Aristotle*, 13.

# 3  EXPLAINING AIDS: A CASE STUDY
## Mary Ann Gardell Cutter

This chapter investigates the ways in which medicine explains the clinical problem known as acquired immunodeficiency syndrome (AIDS) from a philosophical perspective.[1] If successful, it should contribute to one of philosophy's central tasks, namely, to aid an applied science such as medicine in clarifying its ideas, concepts, and values.

In explaining clinical problems, medicine seeks to bring meaning to the ways in which we know and manipulate disease and illness. The medical explanation of AIDS nicely illustrates three important features of this enterprise. First, the more one advances in the process of explaining clinical problems, the more one deals with entities that are human constructions: creatures of thought expressing certain recognizable observables in nature. As an illustration, the first part of this essay discusses the ways in which contemporary medicine has successively explained AIDS in terms of a syndrome, an etiological agent, and a model.[2] The movement through these explanatory levels reflects medicine's effort to know truly and to know effectively, that is, to understand clinical problems in a way that will facilitate their resolution within the life of a particular sociocultural setting. The second section below explores how these epistemic (knowledge-gathering) and nonepistemic (action-oriented) concerns of clinical explanation interact in the explanation of AIDS. Finally, the last section discusses the role that negotiation plays in fashioning clinical explanation by examining in greater detail the ways in which nonepistemic concerns have shaped our understanding of AIDS.

21

## VARYING VISIONS OF AIDS: A CASE STUDY
## IN CLINICAL EXPLANATION

The year 1981 marked the emergence of a medical consensus that a pattern of observable signs and symptoms forecasting nearly inevitable death was occurring in isolated groups in the United States.[3] Signs, such as skin lesions, lymphadenopathy, and unusual infections, and symptoms, such as fatigue, recurrent fevers, unintended weight loss, and uncontrollable diarrhea, were brought together in an organized pattern, or *syndrome*. This syndrome was seen to occur primarily in the four *H* groups, namely, Haitians, hemophiliacs, heroin users, and homosexual males. The majority of cases were appearing in the last group, one composed of individuals viewed as highly "promiscuous."[4] The problem was shown to be acquired rather than inherited.[5] Through the recognition of a collection of signs and symptoms recurring in a specific pattern, acquired immunodeficiency syndrome became a clinical reality. As the AIDS researcher Michael Gottlieb put it, "the third case [of AIDS] clinched the realization that what I was seeing was something new. I knew I was witnessing medical history, but I had no comprehension of what this illness would become."[6] The result was our concept of "clinical AIDS."

The recognition of a syndrome may be considered the first level in our understanding of a clinical problem. At this level, clinical observers have their attention arrested by a pattern of disease phenomena, a characteristic syndrome. By describing "clinical entities," clinicians attempt to make the world intelligible enough to explain. If, in addition, observers notice that certain interventions act effectively to change (that is, to treat) conditions, clinicians then come into possession of an empirical intervention. In the AIDS story, early recommendations on treating a patient's fever and loss of body fluids may be considered a form of clinical maneuvering at this level of syndrome identification. Treatment at the level of syndrome identification, symptomatic treatment, seeks relief of the complaints for which patients come to physicians for help. In symptomatic treatment, physicians have no reason to believe they are addressing some underlying basis of the syndrome.

Syndromes provide the basis for the development of etiological frameworks that allow signs and symptoms to be related in causal terms. During 1983 and 1984, transmissible agents were shown to be responsible for the manifestation and spread of AIDS. Members of a French group headed by Luc Montagnier of the Pasteur Institute first labeled the pathogen they described as the lymphadenopathy-associated virus, or LAV,[7] and later as immune deficiency-associated viruses or IDAVs and finally as lymphadenopathy/AIDS virus, or LAV again.[8] The claim here was that the AIDS virus belonged in the lentivirus family, as it may traverse the blood-brain barrier, resulting in brain damage.

Across the Atlantic, a group in the United States, headed by Robert Gallo of the National Cancer Institute (NCI),[9] identified the AIDS pathogen as human T-cell lymphotropic virus type-III, or HTLV-III. For Gallo and his colleagues, the pathogen appeared to be a mutant of another human T-cell lymphotropic virus, HTLV-I, which caused leukemia by transforming T-cells and causing them to multiply at an excessive rate. HTLV-III was believed to incorporate itself into the T-cells, ultimately destroying them and leaving the organism without immunological protection. The discussions did not end there, for those working with Jay Levy of the University of California at San Francisco offered yet another interpretation of the AIDS virus, naming it AIDS-associated retrovirus (ARV).[10]

The French-U.S. debate illustrates the sociocultural character of medical explanation. Medicine explains clinical problems through communities of individuals mutually exchanging ideas, if not actively challenging each other's evidence and rules of inference.[11] The acrimonious disputes over the French and U.S. findings reflected the beginnings of a shift from viewing the clinical problem as simply a "clinical entity," or pattern (*ens morbi*), to interpreting it in terms of a causal entity that can unify the appearances and make the pattern intelligible (*causi morbi*).[12] The theoretical significance of the shift is justified by its pragmatic force: One can now isolate causes that recommend themselves as mutable variables. One chooses an etiological theory to highlight variables open to easy influence. Thus, clinical AIDS increasingly becomes "HIV disease."

In the AIDS story, the etiological explanation of one form of the syndrome could be used in preventing HIV transmission by testing for HIV antibodies and curtailing certain behavioral (sexual, occupational, drug-related) practices. Future strategies for preventing HIV infection would involve vaccine or specific antiviral therapy. The value of the causal explanation of AIDS, in other words, lay in its ability to spur new developments in the *treatment* of AIDS.[13]

Given an etiological explanation for AIDS, the clinical investigation prepared for the development of a theoretical framework in which all the variables could be related within a nomological (lawlike) structure. The cause of AIDS, though perhaps necessary for the manifestation of the disease, was insufficient to account for it. Montagnier and his colleagues claimed that the AIDS virus shared genetic similarities with viruses in the lentivirus family.[14] U.S. researchers under Max Essex at Harvard argued that the AIDS virus reflected the genetic character of Gallo's leukemia virus.[15] What these views shared was an understanding of AIDS in terms of the multifactorial, as opposed to unifactorial, interplay among the etiological and symptomatic factors associated with the problem. AIDS is conceived in terms of a theory-structure in which all the variables associated with the problem (for example, signs, symptoms) are understood in terms of their causal relatedness.

The possibility of dealing efficiently with clinical problems gives the shift from disease entities to disease models practical importance. Clinical problems are no longer appreciated merely as syndromes or as effects of unifactorial entities, but rather as relations among numerous intervening variables. The possibilities for treating AIDS thus broaden.[16] It may be in certain circumstances that social variables, which presuppose the least technological advance, are easiest to alter. One is reminded here of the campaign of the Centers for Disease Control to alter the behavior of those in AIDS high-risk groups or who associated with people in such groups,[17] or attempts by Matilde Krim to make available sterile, unused hypodermic needles to drug addicts.[18] By allowing the emphasis to fall upon relations, rather than objects or isolated causal agents, medicine conceives of clinical problems in terms that are open to a wide range of purposes.

This brief overview indicates three degrees of abstraction in the development of the explanation of AIDS: as a syndrome, as an etiological account, and as a model. These levels reveal important conceptual legacies that reverberate through present disputes regarding the character of AIDS. Now we may focus, as the next section does, on the ways in which clinical explanation seeks to know the character of clinical problems truly and effectively.

## KNOWING TRULY AND KNOWING EFFECTIVELY IN CLINICAL MEDICINE

In part, clinical explanations reflect clinicians' epistemic interests in knowing truly[19] the character of human disease and illness. In endeavoring to "know truly," clinicians attempt to understand a clinical problem from the viewpoint of a dispassionate observer, so that their findings may be shared with others. Thus epistemic interest is governed by criteria, such as empirical adequacy, statistical relevance, coherence, simplicity, and elegance, that are designed to screen out personal value judgments from clinical explanations. These criteria are reflected, for example, in the medical community's pursuit of the precise genetic structure of the AIDS virus[20] and of a coherent account of the role of T4 cells in the proliferation of the AIDS virus.[21]

This view of the nature of clinical explanation forms the basis of a large body of literature in the philosophy of science and of medicine. It presumes clinical problems to be purely epistemic or rational accounts in which explainers agree on (1) how to acquire evidence relevant to the problem and (2) how to reason with the evidence in order to reach a rationally defensible conclusion that will resolve some question or quandary. This account presents the possibility of a "sound argument" explanation according to a model such as that proposed by Hempel and Oppenheim.[22] With regard to AIDS, one is reminded of the ways in which the Centers for Disease Control explains AIDS on the basis of commonly shared rules of evidence and inference.[23] Such explanations are commonly claimed to be apolitical and impersonal.

In this noncontextual view, it is as if the various political, economic, social, and psychological differences among explainers do not matter. Instead, the participants become anonymous reasoners. In terms of such a view, a final and true explanation should be available to answer the question of why AIDS occurs.

One might argue, however, that clinical explanation is more complex. The rules for acquiring evidence and drawing conclusions in medicine are tied to the ways in which clinical problems are treated. Clinicians' concerns to treat effectively and to act prudently serve to guide the gathering of clinical knowledge. In addition, the rules for inference and evidence change over time. One must, as a consequence, identify a clinical explanation with a particular clinical community, its rules for selecting evidence relevant to an explanation, and its rules for reasoning on the basis of such evidence. Particular clinical communities are merely groups of individual explainers who at a particular point in history share common rules of evidence and inference. As a result, the generation of clinical explanations is subject to the sociopolitical forces that accompany any human community. Even when clinical explanations are somewhat shielded from sociopolitical forces external to the medical community, there are still the community's own internal dynamics to be taken into account. Nonepistemic (that is, action-oriented) considerations thus play an important role in fashioning clinical explanations.

Nonepistemic influences in clinical explanations encompass a wide range of considerations, including cost-benefit, economic, political, and legal concerns, that are tied to the ways clinical problems are manipulated and controlled. One can appreciate the role nonepistemic interests play in clinical explanations when one considers the ways in which accounts of AIDS function as treatment warrants. To construe AIDS as a genetic, infectious, immunological, or behavioral problem radically alters the direction of treatment. Whether one treats AIDS with a vaccine or specific antiviral drug or by curtailing certain behavioral practices will turn on one's interpretations of the problem. Our understanding of AIDS is altered as well by sociopolitical forces. One might consider the French-U.S. debates on the nature of the AIDS virus, especially with regard to the controversy over which group should receive the benefits to be derived from isolating the AIDS virus.[24] At stake here are questions regarding whether the U.S. government or the Pasteur Institute is entitled to the patent rights on kits that are being used commercially to test blood samples for antibodies to the AIDS virus. Sociopolitical forces thus shape the character of clinical explanations by influencing the views of participants, the selection of treatments, and the allocation of perquisites, power, and economic advantages.

Nonepistemic considerations enter, then, into the ways in which clinical explanations are fashioned. Clinical explanation is marked by value-infectedness and culture-relativity not simply because of the ways in which values and culture adventitiously influence knowledge claims but because values and cultural interests are an integral part of medicine as an applied science. Though they may be distinguished, then, epistemic concerns are inseparable from nonepistemic ones. Knowing truly is tied inextricably to knowing effectively.

## NEGOTIATING THE WAYS OF CLINICAL EXPLANATION

The more clinical medicine frames explanations that are open to a wide range of influences, the more it is necessary to have *common* understandings of the significance and consequences of employing clinical explanations as warrants for action. Clinical explanation requires acting as if a particular account (for example, of the nature of the AIDS virus) is correct. However, the choice of any particular clinical explanation carries particular social costs. Deciding that one viral model accounts for the causal agent of AIDS while another form does not will mean relying more heavily on some studies rather than on others. Here, one is reminded of the dispute over the naming of the AIDS virus.[25] Choices must be made concerning which group of studies to rely on. These studies included, as Harold Varmus indicates,[26] those engaged in by individuals claiming recognition in the discovery of AIDS (for example, Essex, Gallo, Levy, Montagnier). The choice of some studies over others necessarily left out other potential candidates to this claim to fame. Furthermore, the naming of the AIDS virus turned on decisions regarding what accords with proper taxonomic design, what would be most acceptable to those working with actual AIDS patients in the clinic, and what would be least biased in favoring one interpretation of the causative agent over another. The naming of the AIDS virus was thus fraught with scientific, social, and political considerations. Only out of this process did the AIDS virus acquire its new name: human immunodeficiency virus, or HIV.

In addition, the selection of a clinical explanation as correct or good will turn on the basis of the costs of being wrong. One can fail, for instance, to make acceptable cost-benefit, risk-benefit, or harm-benefit determinations. In much of clinical explanation, there is a considerable risk that acting on a faulty explanation will mean instituting the wrong treatment. To decide on the costs of various mistakes, one must weigh the costs of treatment for diseases the patient does not in fact have against the cost of not treating afflicted patients.[27] In the case of AIDS, if one adopts standards for treatment that are too lax, one may unduly increase the economic, social, and personal costs of care for individuals as well as the collective whole.[28] However, if one sets the standards too strictly, one will pay the cost in loss of lives. As a consequence, one must decide upon a prudent balancing of the risks of over- versus underexplaining costly results.

Such assessments require a prior comparison of the various possible benefits and harms involved in the clinical choices at hand. However, there is unlikely to be initial agreement with respect to such rank orderings. The results are often clinical explanations with heavy political and ethical overlays. For example, consider the controversies surrounding the determination of the proper standards for exposure to the AIDS virus in the clinical setting[29] and the workplace.[30] Such explanations of the ways in which HIV is transmitted from individual to individual turn on varying views of what counts as proper scientific evidence and rules of inference and of what risks we are willing to take in order to save lives in occupational settings. Points of disagreement are likely to be multiple and intricate.

In resolving disputes about how best to explain a clinical problem, it will be impossible to appeal to a disinterested rational observer in order to acquire a single best answer. This ideal is simply unattainable. In explaining AIDS one is not simply describing genetic-pathological functioning. One is accounting for a clinical problem in terms of a wide range of nonepistemic factors. One is forced to choose among various interpretations, to act on some of them, and eventually to pay the consequences of possible misjudgment. Clinical explanations of AIDS are, in short, contextual.

As the foregoing suggests, there is no single answer to the question of how AIDS is explained. Clinical explanation is a heterogeneous and complex endeavor, appealing to a wide range of epistemic and nonepistemic considerations. As a creative process, clinical explanation requires continued negotiation among those concerned in order to elucidate the character of a particular clinical problem. This chapter, along with the others in this volume, contributes to the process of elucidating the ways by which we seek through explanation to know the character of AIDS both truly and effectively.

## NOTES

1. By "explain" I mean an act that explicates the relation among sets of evidence in some rationally defensible fashion, thus resolving some question or dispute. By "medicine" I mean a heterogeneous and complex discipline embracing a range of goals, including understanding human disease and illness; secur-

ing freedom from pain; maintaining, preserving, and restoring bodily form and certain human abilities; and postponing or preparing for an unacceptable death. By "clinical problem" I mean conditions that warrant the attention of medical practitioners. Such a term refers usually to conditions that are considered causally determined (that is, not directly or immediately under voluntary control) and that are recognized as the substrata of dysfunctions, pains, or disfigurements.

2. H. T. Engelhardt, Jr. Explanatory models in medicine: Facts, theories, and values. *Texas Reports in Biology and Medicine* 56 (1974):225–39.

3. Centers for Disease Control. Pneumocystis pneumonia—Los Angeles. *Morbidity and Mortality Weekly Reports* 30 (1981):250–52.

4. Centers for Disease Control. Kaposi's sarcoma and pneumocystis pneumonia among homosexual men—New York City and California. *Morbidity and Mortality Weekly Reports* 30 (1981):305–8.

5. R. M. Selik, H. W. Haverkos, and J. W. Curren. Acquired immune deficiency syndrome (AIDS) trends in the United States, 1978–1982. *American Journal of Medicine* 76 (1984):493–500.

6. M. Gottlieb. Quoted in C. Wallis. AIDS: A growing threat. *Time* 126 (1985): 41.

7. J. E. Conte. Infection-control guidelines for patients with acquired immunodeficiency syndrome. *New England Journal of Medicine* 309 (1983):740–44.

8. F. Barre-Sinoussi et al. Isolation of T-lymphotropic retrovirus from a patient at risk for acquired immunodeficiency syndrome (AIDS). *Science* 220 (1983):868–71.

9. R. C. Gallo et al. Frequent detection and isolation of cytopathic retroviruses (HTLV-III) from patients with AIDS and at risk for AIDS. *Science* 224 (1984):500–3.

10. J. A. Levy et al. Isolation of lymphocytopathic retroviruses from San Francisco patients with AIDS. *Science* 225 (1984):840–42.

11. L. Fleck. *Genesis and Development of a Scientific Fact*, trans. F. Bradley and T. J. Trenn. Chicago: University of Chicago Press, 1981. First published 1935.

12. H. T. Englehardt, Jr. Typologies of disease: nosologies revisited. In *Logic in Discovery and Diagnosis in Medicine*, ed. K. Schaffner. Berkeley: University of California Press, 1985, pp. 56–71.

13. J. W. Curren et al. The epidemiology of AIDS: Current status and future prospects. *Science* 229 (1985):1352–57.

14. F. Clavel et al. Isolation of a new human retrovirus from West African patients with AIDS. *Science* 233 (1986):343–46.

15. P. Boffey. U.S. and French teams report AIDS virus findings. *New York Times* (March 16, 1986): 1, 7.

16. Office of Technology Assessment. *Review of the Public Health Service's Response to AIDS*. Washington, D.C.: U.S. Government Printing Office, 1985.

17. Centers for Disease Control. Classification system for human T-lymphotropic virus type III/lymphadenopathy-associated virus infections. *Morbidity and Mortality Weekly Reports* 35 (1986):19–23.

18. M. Krim. AIDS: The challenge to science and medicine. *Hastings Center Report* 15 (August 1985):2–7.

19. E. McMullin. Scientific controversy and its termination. In *Scientific Controversies*, ed. H. T. Engelhardt, Jr., and A. Caplan. Cambridge: Cambridge University Press, 1987, pp. 49–91.

20. F. Wong-Staal et al. Genome diversity of human T-lymphotropic virus type III (HTLV-III). *Science* 229 (1985):750–62.

21. R. S. Kalish and S. F. Schossman. The T4 lymphocyte in AIDS. *New England Journal of Medicine* 313 (1985):112–13.

22. C. Hempel and P. Oppenheim. Studies in the logic of explanation. *Philosophy of Science* 15 (1948):135–78.

23. Centers for Disease Control. Update: Acquired immunodeficiency syndrome—United States. *Morbidity and Mortality Weekly Reports* 35 (1986):17–21.

24. C. Norman. Patent dispute divides AIDS researchers. *Science* 230 (1985): 640–42; C. Norman. A new twist in AIDS patent fight. *Science* 232 (1986):308–9.

25. J. Coffin et al. Human immunodeficiency viruses. *Science* 232 (1986):697.

26. H. E. Varmus. Naming the AIDS virus. This volume, Chapter 1.

27. H. T. Engelhardt, Jr. *The Foundations of Bioethics*. New York: Oxford University Press, 1986.

28. A. M. Hardy et al. The economic impact of the first 10,000 cases of acquired immunodeficiency syndrome in the United States. *Journal of the American Medical Association* 255 (1986):209–15.

29. E. McCray et al. Occupational risk of the acquired immunodeficiency syndrome among health care workers. *New England Journal of Medicine* 314 (1986): 1127–32.

30. M. Sande. The case against casual transmission. *New England Journal of Medicine* 314 (1986):380–82.

# 4 ETHICS AND THE LANGUAGE OF AIDS
*Judith Wilson Ross*

> If names are not correct, language is not in accordance with the truth
> of things. If language is not in accordance with the truth of things,
> affairs cannot be carried on to success.
>
> Confucian Analects, Book XIII

AIDS has proved a difficult phenomenon medically, but it is equally
problematic from a linguistic perspective. As many writers have commented, the problems that AIDS presents appear new to us because very
few remember the great influenza epidemic of 1918–19 and not many
have more than dim memories of the pre-1944 fear of tuberculosis or of
the relatively small polio epidemics of the 1930s and 1940s. For the most
part, we have spent our lives in a culture in which infectious disease
does not represent a significant threat and we have consigned living in
fear of life-threatening contagious disease to the pages of history books.
New phenomena, however, whether they are new in cultural or in personal history, demand descriptions and explanations. The language in
which we choose to describe new phenomena displays both the context
and the meaning we give to them. In particular, the metaphors we use
convey much of the deeper meaning that we attribute to these new
events.

Public policy, ethical judgments, and personal choices can all be deeply influenced by the metaphors we have chosen or have grown accustomed to using and hearing others use. We may talk of facts and objective judgments, but facts can be arranged in many ways to prove many

things. They are not as immutable as the scientists would have us believe. Scientific facts, beyond the abstractions of pure mathematics, cannot long exist, as independent entities are soon transformed into the linguistic patterns of everyday use, where decision-making takes place. Thus, the language of AIDS not only reveals how we perceive the disease, but also directly influences public decisions and private behavior by providing implicit justifications for our choices. In this paper, I examine the metaphors for AIDS—death, sin, crime, war, and civic division—which are the shaping perceptions that make the language of AIDS so dangerous.

## THE DEATH METAPHOR

AIDS is perhaps first of all a metaphor of personified death. The personal account literature is full of references to people who "lost" lovers or friends to AIDS. "AIDS took three people on this street," an acquaintance told me. A young man with AIDS says, "Why did it get me?" In *Life* magazine, "AIDS struck the Burk family," and it "laid their bodies open to lethal infections."[1] Here, AIDS becomes powerful and independent. It goes about choosing its victims, a grim reaper hiding behind ordinary sexual relationships. In *Rolling Stone*,[2] Edmund White uses this metaphor quite specifically: "Gay sex has become equated with death. Behind the friendly smiling face, bronzed and mustachioed, is a skull. . . . " The ubiquitous use of the word "victim" is part of the *AIDS as Death* metaphor. Death in our culture is not a kindly God looking to bring his people back into his presence. It is a skeletal figure, stealing people and taking them into the realm of darkness. AIDS is Death out looking for victims.

This image of AIDS as Death is reinforced throughout the popular and quasi-academic literature by the unrelenting joining of the word AIDS with the phrase "inevitably/invariably fatal." It is as if one expected a diagnosis of AIDS to lead to instant death. Yet, many people with AIDS live on for months or even years and live for the most part outside the hospital. The metaphor of AIDS as Death permits us to forget those who have the syndrome: They are dead to us, making it easier to withhold both aggressive treatment and financial assistance.

Here, scientific information could help to straighten out our metaphor. From a medical perspective, AIDS is considered to be "invariably fatal" only because it has, historically, been defined that way.[3] When the Centers for Disease Control (CDC) provided its definition for surveillance purposes, little was known about the natural history of the disease. Now, years later, it is obvious that AIDS is not an isolated disease or even a disease syndrome. CDC maintains its definition for the limited purposes of epidemiological surveillance, although the definition is not accurate for other purposes.[4] The clinical disease is obviously one small part of a spectrum of diseases caused by infection with HIV. Its effects range from a brief and transient illness, through generalized lymphadenopathy, to what is called AIDS-related complex (ARC), and on to frank or full-blown AIDS. Robert Gallo and other scientists have argued for change in this nomenclature.[5] Yet, we cling to AIDS as Death, to AIDS as an invariably fatal disease, perhaps because it better fits the drama that we have constructed about the coming of and meaning of AIDS.

## THE PUNISHMENT METAPHOR

The metaphor of AIDS as Death leads directly to the metaphor of AIDS as punishment for sin. If Death is about, looking for new victims, then the victim inevitably asks, "Why was I chosen?" Those who feel threatened also look to find reasons why they may be protected: They ask, "Why not me?" To answer these questions, the disease is characterized as the result of something over which people have some control, most particularly their own behavior.

Historically, new and threatening events have frequently (some would say invariably) been explained by reference to God's punishment. In the Bible, God repeatedly punishes with disease and with plagues. In Defoe's semifictional account of the 1665 plague, the *Journal of the Plague Year*, he describes the ways in which, at the beginning of the plague, the people looked first to astrologers to explain it as a result of astral doings, then to dream interpreters, and finally to preachers, who explained it in terms of God's judgment, the "dreadful judgment which hung over their heads."[6]

Fundamentalist ministers have been the most constant exponents of this version of AIDS as punishment for sin. Thus, the Moral Majority's Jerry Falwell is reputed to have claimed that "AIDS is the wrath of God upon homosexuals."[7] Other fundamentalist ministers have been as forthright in their claims.[8] More ecumenically, the Anglican dean of Sydney, Australia, is quoted as saying that "gays have blood on their hands."[9] In a secular vein, President Reagan's speechwriter Pat Buchanan has written that "the poor homosexuals have declared war on nature and now nature is exacting an awful retribution."[10] Although cleansed of religious implications, this is the same view of AIDS as punishment for sin, but here sin is seen as a violation of the natural law rather than as a violation of God's law. A variation of this metaphor appears in the account of the young man with AIDS who promises his doctor that, if he recovers, he will get a girlfriend.[11] This is sin followed by penance.

It is easy to dismiss that kind of talk as merely the babblings of exceedingly small-minded souls or minds overstressed by illness, and yet the metaphor of AIDS as punishment for sin flourishes as well in academic and liberal forums. AIDS is transmitted sexually and through the blood. Two behaviors statistically account for 90 percent of these transmissions in the United States: homosexual intercourse and illegal intravenous (IV) drug use. Both these behaviors are regarded as sinful by many and perhaps most people: In the United States, gay sex is still illegal in half of the states, and IV drug use without a prescription is illegal in all states. Because behavior that is regarded as sinful has resulted in exposure to disease, it is easy for the disease to become the punishment for the sin.

Thus, James L. Fletcher, in an editorial in the *Southern Medical Journal,* cautioned that "a logical conclusion is that AIDS is a self-inflicted disorder for the majority of those who suffer from it. . . . Perhaps then, homosexuality is not 'alternative' behavior at all, but, as the ancient wisdom of the Bible states, most certainly pathologic." He concludes by suggesting that physicians would do well to seek "reversal treatment" for their gay patients.[12] Similarly, Joseph Perloff, professor of medicine at the University of California at Los Angeles, denies that there is any scapegoating going on with AIDS because "it is not correct to say that nobody is to blame. . . . Ninety percent of all AIDS cases are contracted by either specific sexual acts or specific IV drug abuse. The remaining 10 percent—recipients of blood transfusions, children of female AIDS patients, hemophiliacs—may well be regarded as mere 'victims.'"[13]

The overflow of this metaphor is seen in the insistence on promiscuity as the source of AIDS. Matt Herron, writing in *The Whole Earth Review* in an article that is clearly not intended to be punitive toward gays, nevertheless comments that when "AIDS arrived, . . . the doors of the candy store started to close." Gays, in his account, had been feasting on forbidden sweets and AIDS was a predictable result of this excess. AIDS was not just a disease in this account, nor even *merely* personal punishment for sin. According to Herron, "the teaching of AIDS," is that "[if you] mess around on a grand enough scale, you will begin to disturb human biology itself."[14]

In the general medical literature, writers frequently refer to promiscuity as the source of AIDS, easily confusing a statistical phenomenon with a judgmental one. Even if they were genuinely trying only to indicate that having an increased number of sexual partners heightens the risk of having a partner who carries the virus, the choice of the word "promiscuity" is suspect. "Promiscuous" carries with it a moral judgment; it does not simply mean having multiple sexual partners. Promiscuous, in the context of the nation's sexual nervousness, very probably means having more sexual partners than the speaker currently has, that is, an inappropriate or morally reprehensible number.[15] Incorporating this word into serious general or medical writing is probably far more effective than Falwell and Buchanan could ever hope to be in driving home the message that AIDS is punishment for sin.

The gay press also has writers in this vein. Ned Rorem, writing in *The Advocate*, a national gay journal, wonders whether (with respect to AIDS) "some chastisement is at work."[16] Writers who are encouraging reduced numbers of sexual relationships for gay men are now beginning to make a virtue of this reduction, so that monogamy is seen as a morally correct gay lifestyle. Although monogamy will statistically reduce one's chances of coming in contact with HIV, that in itself is certainly no endorsement of the moral splendor of monogamy or even of its safety, if one's single partner happens to be carrying the virus. Yet, the metaphor of AIDS as punishment for sin makes the designation of gay monogamy as a virtue seem to be correct.[17]

A final way in which AIDS as punishment for sin is foisted upon us is in the idea of "innocent victims." "Innocence" belongs to the vocabulary of sin. Gay people who never heard of AIDS until they were diagnosed to have it are never referred to as "innocent" nor are IV drug users who encountered HIV entirely to their surprise. *Innocent* victims of AIDS are babies, elderly women, and nuns, all of who are presumed to have led, for a variety of reasons, blameless lives. This labeling of victims as "innocent" and, by indirection, "guilty" is translated into action in hospitals, in public agencies, and in the news media, where gay men or drug users with AIDS are treated with less sympathy than "innocent" AIDS patients, that is, those who have not sinned on their way to illness; those for whom the disease does not represent their just desserts.

## THE CRIME AND CRIMINAL METAPHORS

The AIDS *victim* (guilty *or* innocent) also belongs to the metaphor of AIDS as crime. It is almost impossible to find an article in the popular press about people with AIDS that does not use the word "victim" several times. When Los Angeles Archbishop Mahoney announced that the diocese intended to open a hospice for those with AIDS, he could scarcely get through a sentence without talking about "victims." In an interchange that particularly demonstrated the strained use of language, he finally declared, when asked if the hospice would be open only to Catholics, that it would indeed be open to "victims of any faith or belief."[18]

The use of the word "victim" can, of course, create sympathy for those with AIDS, but it can also make them feel helpless. In addition, when those with AIDS are portrayed as victims, it is because they have had something unexpected done to them, something that is somehow against the law, if only the scientific law as we imaginatively perceive it. Thus, AIDS becomes a supercriminal able to get away with violating the law. It is seen as amazing, Lex Luthor-like, someone who sweeps across the world, striking terror in people's hearts. *Newsweek* describes AIDS "embark[ing] on an intercontinental killing spree." It becomes a serial killer that "strikes men and women" and "makes deep incursions on heterosexuals."[19] It goes on "a deadly odyssey."[20]

For the *Los Angeles Times*, AIDS becomes a "pathological personality."[21] This language presents a disease that is larger than life. Its power is awesome, and we can only be terrified by it. This kind of image can be used to encourage increased spending (it's so big that you need to spend a lot of money to control it), but it also encourages drastic steps, steps that go outside the ordinary bounds of good sense, good law, and good ethics. Discussions about quarantine often interpret AIDS this way. The battle over closing the bathhouses may have been affected by this draconian aspect of the crime-criminal metaphor because although many acknowledged the closing to be a drastic action, it could be justified by the enormity of the "criminal" that was being tracked.

In addition to appearing as a master criminal, AIDS also appears as a new kind of crime. New diseases are easily seen in a crime metaphor exactly because we do not understand them. They then present themselves as puzzles or as mysteries. "An unidentified disease mysteriously focuses on one group."[22] This metaphor feeds directly into our rather trivial fantasies about detective stories and turns physician-scientists into detectives scrambling about, using their superior intellectual abilities to unravel the mystery. It makes "unravelling the secrets of the shifty AIDS virus" the important aspect, not the care of those with the disease. Indeed, it tends to reduce those who actually have the disease to objects from which useful information can be sought: a source of new clues. In a recent issue of the *New York Times Magazine*, there is a colorful account of the work of four Boston physicians and researchers who are presented as a crackerjack, coordinated, and collaborative detective team out to solve the mystery.[23] The detective story metaphor is widely apparent in the popular press: The *Philadelphia Daily News* warns of a "Gay Plague baffling medical detectives."[24] "Clues" turn up everywhere. *Medical World News* advises its readers that "mounting evidence suggests that . . . heterosexuals may find themselves tangled in the AIDS web."[25]

The primary problem with the detective story metaphor is that it tends to confound the *disease* as crime and criminal with the *person who has the disease* as crime and criminal. Thus, whereas *Newsweek* describes AIDS as terrorizing the world, *Life* magazine asserts that "the AIDS *minorities* are beginning to infect the heterosexual, drug-free majority"[26] and *Weekly World News*, moving one step further, proclaims: "AIDS *victims* terrorizing everybody"[27] [emphasis added].

## THE WAR METAPHOR

The metaphor of medicine as war is so common that we can scarcely imagine any other way of talking about how physicians deal with diseases and patients. The physicians' job is, after all, to fight disease. They use batteries of tests and have an armamentarium of drugs. They give orders. Their troops, of course, owe them obedience and loyalty. This metaphor developed first in the late nineteenth century with the discovery of bacteria, which were seen as invaders.[28] HIV infection, as a disease that effects the immune system (with its killer cells that fight off foreign invaders) is particularly surrounded by a scientific vocabulary based on war metaphors. For example, one writer explains that "when the battle against the invading microorganisms is done, . . . T-suppressor cells send out signals to call off the troops." When the AIDS virus appears, it "must first invade a host cell and commandeer some of that cell's DNA material." Eventually, "the body is completely at the mercy of the most commonplace of infectious invaders."[29]

AIDS as a war ("The AIDS Conflict," according to *Newsweek*[30]) is reported much as any other war is. Intrepid *Cosmopolitan* reporter Ralph Gardner, Jr., advises his readers that "if this is a battle that pits man against nature, then nature is pushing back our forces. The news from the front is not good."[31] A dedicated rallier of the troops, Detroit physician John F. Fennessey, does not take such news lying down. He issues a clarion call that "AIDS must be confronted, attacked, and bested by the full, coordinated resources and armamentarium of the medical scientific community. . . . AIDS must and will be confronted and controlled."[32]

Although much of this sounds like no more than bad writing, it is important to remember that the primary element of the war metaphor is the existence of an enemy. AIDS or HIV is, presumably, that enemy. As the crime metaphor permits the person who has the disease to become the criminal, so also does the war metaphor encourage transforming the person housing the enemy into the enemy. Thus, *Medical World News* reports that "an infected person could harbor the virus for 14.2 years."[33] *Life* refers to the 1.3 million people in the United States who "may be harboring—and passing on—the virus without having symptoms."[34]

Outside of ship anchorage, "harbor" is probably most closely associated with spies and criminals (as in harboring criminals or spies). Harboring suggests that the virus is being hidden knowingly, willingly, and with bad intentions. It does not regard the "infected person" as a neutral object. In a war, those who "harbor" the virus are like spies in our midst. Demands for quarantine and isolation of those with AIDS or for labeling and tracking asymptomatic people who are antibody positive are calls to locate the enemy. They are reminiscent of World War II internment policies that we now look back upon with great discomfort. No one believed that *all* Japanese residents were a threat to the country but, since the dangerous ones could not be identified, it seemed appropriate to incarcerate all of them. This decision was supported by the public and, ultimately, by the U.S. Supreme Court because it occurred in the context of a great war. To the extent that the war metaphor dominates our perceptions of AIDS, we will be more likely to sacrifice people and their rights in the name of protecting society. Edmund White, writing in *Rolling Stone*, argues that "gays are quickly losing basic civil liberties. A real state of siege has been declared."[35] Clearly the war has been declared not on the virus but upon those who carry it.

The war metaphor also gives rise to other elaborations. Susan Sontag has commented that writing about cancer is so dominated by war metaphors that the only thing missing is the body count.[36] Newspaper articles on AIDS now routinely include that body count. The last paragraph of news stories almost invariably gives the absolutely up-to-date number of cases and deaths. A scientist calls asymptomatic, antibody-positive individuals "time bomb[s]" because doctors are unsure of when they will "go off," that is, develop disease.[37] AIDS itself is a "time bomb," according to the *Los Angeles Times*, because of its financial implications.[38] Bombs loom increasingly large. Several writers, including John Brennan (a *Los Angeles Times* medical columnist), have called for a "Manhattan Project" to fight the "war against AIDS."[39] Brennan even goes so far as to say that creating an AIDS Manhattan Project will produce in a short time the necessary weapons (that is, drugs and vaccines) to win the war, just as the original Manhattan Project, in only three years, created the atomic bomb, thus "marking the beginning of the use and abuse of nuclear power." The hope of controlling AIDS with something even metaphorically like the atomic bomb is scarcely an encouraging prospect, especially if we must think of it in terms of the abuse of nuclear power. Brennan's statement shows how easily the war metaphor draws one to otherwise unacceptable ideas.

## THE METAPHOR OF OTHERNESS: THE DIVIDED COMMUNITY

The most difficult metaphor to illustrate in the language of AIDS may be the most pervasive one. That is the language of *otherness*, of the divided community. It is heard easily in conversation. Ask half a dozen people what is to be done about the problem of asymptomatic but infectious seropositives and the usual response is in terms of what "we" must do about "them." The image of AIDS has been carefully sustained as a problem for "them," whoever they may be. Margaret Heckler publicly illustrated this when she announced the availability of the HIV antibody blood test, saying that "we must conquer [AIDS] as well before it . . .

threatens the health of our general population."[40] There was considerable distress expressed about this statement, especially from the gay community, who thought they were a part of the general public. Nevertheless, the phrase continues to be used in discussions about whether AIDS risk groups will change.[41] The speakers seem to believe that they can move the threat of disease further away by casting the high-risk groups out, as if a linguistic distance might provide physical safety.

The persistent recurrence of "leper" and "leprosy" in AIDS discussions and writings is also a part of this metaphor. Lepers are cast out; they are no longer an integral part of the community. Omnipresent analogies between AIDS and leprosy make it seem acceptable to respond to the newer "plague" in the same way that was acceptable for the older one.

The metaphor of AIDS as otherness permits people to accept less treatment for those who belong to that other group than they would demand for themselves. Gardner, for example, points out that "if there was any good news . . . it was only that the great majority of cases (94 percent) remain confined to the four high-risk groups."[42] The idea of otherness is possible only as long as "we" are able to isolate ourselves from linguistic connection with people who have the disease or who are at risk for it. By referring in print to AIDS as a "gay disease" or a "gay plague," those in the straight community are encouraged to think of AIDS as something happening beyond their borders, outside the "general population," people for whom they have no human responsibility. The metaphor of otherness provides comfort to those who use it because it implies that they will be spared harm and responsibility.

## CONCLUSION

In The Plague—Camus's penetrating novel of the way in which the residents of the town of Oran, quarantined with bubonic plague, come to grips with their fate—Tarrou tells Dr. Rieux what he thinks must be done. Through the months, he says, "I'd come to realize that all our troubles spring from our failure to use plain, clean-cut language. So I resolved always to speak—and to act—quite clearly, as this was the only way of setting myself on the right track."[43] Susan Sontag, in a much different context, echoes this statement when she argues that "the most truthful way of regarding illness—and the healthiest way of being ill—is one most purified of, most resistant to, metaphoric thinking."[44]

In Camus's tale, the plague creates community where there had been none: "No longer were there individual destinies; only a collective destiny, made of plague and the emotions shared by all." The metaphors of AIDS, however, work in direct opposition to this sense of community. Crime, sin, war, and the divided polity are all metaphors that oppose a sense of community. They are inherently divisive metaphors that suggest we are *not* all in this together. But surely, we are. There is no question but that ethically one ought not to harm innocent persons. But in this situation, we are all innocent. Those who are carriers of the HIV virus need to care about and to protect those who are not. Those who have not been exposed also need to care for and to protect whose who have. It is not that some of "us" need protection and some of "them" need to sacrifice their rights; that some belong to death while others embrace life; that some are righteous and others are sinners; that some are criminals and others their victims; that some are enemies and others loyal and deserving citizens; that some may be cast out, while others are kept securely within. Surely those who have been exposed to AIDS have enough to bear without the additional burdens of these metaphors.

Disease, especially disease that may lead to death, takes on a dramatic quality in this culture. Drama encourages elevated language. A brief stroll through the *Reader's Guide* listing under AIDS will demonstrate the drama that AIDS has provided for readers in the past few years.[45] It is time, however, to speak plainly. There is too much at stake to permit rhetorical flourish to drive our pens. Again quoting Sontag, "nothing is more punitive than to give a disease a meaning—that meaning being invariably a moral one."[46] AIDS has been permitted and encouraged to carry a moral meaning, but that morality is in our minds, not in the disease. If our ethical judgments are not to be based on punitiveness and further divisiveness, it is time for us to confront the inner meanings our language betrays and then to rid not only our speaking and writing but also our thinking of these metaphors and their insidious implications.

## NOTES

1. *Life* (July 1985):12.

2. E. White. The story of the year. *Rolling Stone* (December 19, 1985–January 2, 1986).

3. Dennis Altman also makes this point: "Although people suffering from ARC can be very sick, relatively few go on to develop the full syndrome and die; one wonders whether the media reaction and resulting hysteria would have been noticeably less had the range of less serious illnesses been included in the conceptualization of AIDS itself from the beginning." *AIDS in the Mind of America.* New York: Anchor/Doubleday, 1986, p. 36.

4. See also the Walter Reed staging classification for HTLV-III/LAV infection. [*New England Journal of Medicine* 314 (1985):131–32], in which Redfield et al. create a scale and nomenclature for infection: "the clinical presentation of patients with HTLV-III infections can range from asymptomatic (with viremia or antibody or both), through chronic generalized lymphadenopathy, to sub-clinical and clinical T-cell deficiency" (p. 131).

5. *American Medical News* (January 10, 1986):36. See also D. Dassey. AIDS and testing for AIDS. *Journal of the American Medical Association* 255 (1986):743.

6. D. Defoe. *Journal of the Plague Year*. New York: New Meridien Classics, 1984, p. 36.

7. Falwell has denied this, although several newspaper reporters have insisted that they heard him say it. See Altman, *AIDS*, 67.

8. See, for example, Charles Stanley, president of the Southern Baptist convention, who has said that "AIDS is God indicating his displeasure toward a sinful life style," as quoted in the *Los Angeles Times* (January 24, 1986):5 (sec. 2).

9. Altman, *AIDS*, 25.

10. As quoted in *Newsweek* (August 12, 1985), from *New York Post* (May 24, 25, 1983).

11. Altman, *AIDS*, 17.

12. J. L. Fletcher, editorial, *Southern Medical Journal* 77 (1984):150.

13. *Los Angeles Times* (March 14, 1986):4 (sec. 2).

14. M. Herron. Living with AIDS. *Whole Earth Review* 48 (1985):52.

15. A recent "Dear Abby" included a letter from a woman who "accepted as due punishment" contracting herpes during a period of "promiscuity." She asks "what are the facts regarding formerly promiscuous women and AIDS. How many years must I fear retribution for that phase of my life? And how would you define promiscuous?" Abby's replay is that disease isn't punishment but that anyone "who has a sexual relationship with more than one person at a time is promiscuous." *Los Angeles Times* (March 9, 1986):sec. 6.

16. *The Advocate* (September 19, 1983).

17. Another variation of AIDS as punishment for sin is expressed by Joan McKenna, a "renegade scientist," who tells gays that "you can't *catch* the deficiencies of an impaired immune system. You have to create them." McKenna teaches "thermobaric therapy," which involves cooling the body's "core temperature." *East West Journal* 16 (1986):44.

18. *Los Angeles Times* (February 3, 1986):1 (sec. 2).

19. *Newsweek* (August 12, 1985).

20. *New York Times Magazine* (February 6, 1986):28.

21. *Los Angeles Times* (November 25, 1985):2 (sec. 1).

22. Herron, *Living with AIDS*, 35.

23. *New York Times Magazine* (March 2, 1986). See also Disease Detectives Tracking the Killers: the AIDS Hysteria. *Time* (July 15, 1985).

24. August 9, 1982, 1.

25. *Medical World News* (May 13, 1985):11.

26. *Life* (July 1985):12.

27. (November 26, 1985):35.

28. S. Sontag. *Illness as Metaphor*. New York: Vintage Books, 1979, pp. 64–65.

29. See Herron, *Living with AIDS*, 46.

30. *Newsweek* (September 23, 1985).

31. R. Gardner, Jr. *Cosmopolitan* (November 1984):150, 155–156.

32. AIDS hysteria counterproductive. *American Medical News* (January 17, 1986):4.

33. The AIDS circle widens. *Medical World News* (May 13, 1985):11.

34. *Life* (July 1985).

35. White, The story of the year, 124.

36. Sontag, *Illness*, 64.

37. *American Medical News* (November 22, 1985):28.

38. *Los Angeles Times* (January 12, 1986).

39. *Los Angeles Times* (October 15, 1985):1, 3 (View sec.). An assistant secretary of health told President Reagan that AIDS research was the "health equivalent of the Manhattan project." *Los Angeles Times* (December 20, 1985):2 (sec. 1).

40. As quoted in *Journal of the American Medical Association* 253 (1985):3377.

41. "IV drug users are most responsible for introducing AIDS into the general population." See Herron, *Living with AIDS*, 47. "So far, the epidemiological evidence suggests that the disease hasn't yet spread widely in the general population." C. Marwick. AIDS associated virus yields data to intensifying scientific scrutiny. *Journal of the American Medical Association* 254 (1985):2867. A Washington, D.C., lobbyist is quoted by *American Medical News* as saying that "the federal government recognizes that AIDS is a public health crisis that has the potential for infecting the general population" (January 10, 1986):9.

42. Gardner, *Cosmopolitan* (November 1984):150.

43. A. Camus. *The Plague*. New York: Random House, 1972, p. 236.

44. Sontag, *Illness*, 5–6.

45. "Fatal, incurable, and spreading"; "Battling AIDS"; "The Plague Years"; "AIDS Neglect"; "AIDS Panic"; "Public Enemy #1"; "Death after Sex"; "Homosexual Plague Strikes New Victims"; etc.

46. Sontag, *Illness*, 57.

# 5 MAKING CONTACT: THE AIDS PLAYS
*Joseph Cady and*
*Kathryn Montgomery Hunter*

One of literature's distinctions and benefits is the concrete and individual form it gives to ethical principles and dilemmas that in other discourse
can remain elusively abstract. With its ancient roots as a shared, communal experience, drama especially may provide a vivid and concrete em-
bodiment of a general phenomenon preoccupying an entire society. It
encourages a more pointed awareness of that reality through the personal, intimate contact it offers its audience. Our subject in this chapter is
the different ways in which the two most prominent recent U.S. plays
about AIDS, William M. Hoffman's *As Is* and Larry Kramer's *The Normal
Heart*, attempt to bring us into contact with a physical and moral disaster
we might otherwise repress or ignore.

*As Is*, which opened in New York in March 1985, and *The Normal Heart*,
which premiered in the same city in the following month, were not the
first contemporary plays to focus on AIDS. They were preceded by Jeff
Hagedorn's *One*, a one-person show about AIDS performed in several
smaller U.S. cities; Robert Chesley's *Night Sweat*, which ran Off-Off
Broadway in 1983; and the collection of AIDS pieces presented at San
Francisco's Theater Rhinoceros in late 1984 by the group Artists Involved
with Death and Survival.[1] They were followed in late 1985 by the made-
for-television movie *An Early Frost*. Nevertheless, *As Is* and *The Normal
Heart* are the two stage dramas about AIDS best known to audiences,
and both are especially concerned with the personal and social dimensions of the crisis that, as we have said, drama may be an especially apt
vehicle for addressing. Besides responding to the obvious tragedy of the

epidemic, both plays sense the divisiveness in the human community that the AIDS epidemic can create—divisions both within the homosexual world and between the homosexual and heterosexual communities. And, besides obviously working to engage their viewers in actions against the disease, both plays attempt, in quite different ways, to put their audiences in contact with a reality from which other circumstances might spur them to distance themselves.

## THE NORMAL HEART

In its form and much of its content, Larry Kramer's *The Normal Heart* is a traditional protest play—a linear, literal, and polemical presentation of the current AIDS crisis and of the author's views of what must be done about it. The play's intention to teach and to move an audience that it assumes is at some distance from the subject is apparent even before the action begins. The walls of the open set and the walls surrounding the audience are covered with facts. There are the names of those who have died of the disease, a regularly revised morbidity and mortality count; a comparison of the inadequate appropriations by the City of New York with the much more generous funding in San Francisco; a story-count contrasting the meager *New York Times* coverage of AIDS in the first ten months of 1984 with the extensive space that paper devoted to the first Tylenol poisoning; and a quotation from the report "American Jewry During the Holocaust," which is meant to parallel gay inaction about AIDS with the ineffectiveness of the American Jewish Committee with respect to the genocide of European Jews during World War II and the prewar period of Nazi rule in Germany (pp. 19–22).[2] The play's didactic intent and method continue throughout.

Protest art differs from satire in focusing on those who suffer rather than on the villains who cause the suffering, but it shares satire's claim to tell the plain, unvarnished truth: "This is not art," it asserts, "but an unaltered piece of reality." Thus, the linear, literal plot of *The Normal Heart* is part of its design on us. We follow its protagonist, Ned Weeks, as he is educated about AIDS, helps to found (and is then expelled from) an AIDS action organization resembling New York City's Gay Men's Health Crisis, and meets and lives with his first lover, Felix, whom he loses to the disease. But it is Ned's vision, more than his experience, that we are meant to share. *The Normal Heart* never misses an opportunity to impress upon us expanded versions of the information painted on its set and theater walls.

For instance, Ned's visit to Emma, a physician and the play's "second hero," for a checkup quickly turns into a report on the escalation of the disease, the indifference of the *New York Times* and Mayor Edward Koch, the politics of U.S. health care in general, and the perceived abyss of

New York gay politics. Even Ned's and Felix's first-date scene, potentially the most personal (and the most critical of Ned) in the play, features both a speech by Ned, elaborating the Holocaust analogy, and a critical remark by the usually nonpolitical Felix about a gay male world "filled with nothing but casual sex" (p. 53). Perhaps the most striking example of this subordination of the personal to the political is the play's ending. Ned's and Felix's marriage ceremony in the hospital and Felix's immediate death might have been the points at which a playwright concerned with intense private emotion would have stopped. Kramer ends instead with a speech by Ned castigating himself first for not "fighting harder" against the epidemic and then for failing to tell the now-dead Felix about the gay dance he had witnessed at Yale while there as an invited speaker for Gay Week. It was a dance, he proclaims, attended by "six hundred . . . smart, exceptional gay men and women" (p. 123). AIDS is so horrible and the need for action against it is so imperative, *The Normal Heart* seems to say, that to convey the "purely personal" is a luxury; only repeated exhortations, public pronouncements, and a recital of facts will suffice.

This obvious level of the play, which signifies Kramer's understanding of the enormity of the AIDS crisis and his sense of its solution, seems optimistic: It works to awaken its audience and to agitate for change. Yet its form conveys on a more profound level a contradictory pessimism. The high-decible didacticism and the recurringly public focus reveal a distrust, even a dislike, of its audience—just as its action seems deeply to doubt the possibility of substantial moral change. *The Normal Heart* generated much controversy in the New York gay community for its attacks on the early Gay Men's Health Crisis and on the gay male community in general (which it portrays as overwhelmingly sex obsessed). It was condemned as well for what was seen as its excessive puritanism and for posing a popular "promiscuous" gay male lifestyle against its demand for chastity, even total celibacy. At some point this may have seemed like alarmist common sense, but Emma's repeated dictum that "gay men . . . stop having sex" (p. 37)—even once forbidding kissing—clearly ignores the guidelines for "safe sex" that had already been published by the time of the production.

Although *The Normal Heart* urges connection between lovers, brothers, friends, political allies, and doctor and patient it does not imagine a world where this is possible for long. It is true that by the end of *The Normal Heart* the remaining members of the AIDS action group have their long-awaited meeting with the mayor, that Ned and his heterosexual brother have embraced, and that Ned and Felix are "married." But Ned is excluded from the mayor's meeting, a fact that suggests the meeting will be futile, and death not only ends the marriage but has licensed it. Only Ned's reconciliation with his brother offers hope of contact, and it is a bridge principally for the play's heterosexual audience. These failed or partial connections reveal the play's underlying pessimism. Not only is AIDS unstopped, but Ned and Emma, the play's two heroes, are in their different ways left as "alone against the world" as they were at the play's beginning: Emma, the activist physician who has pioneered in caring for AIDS patients, has had her funding denied by the National Institute of Health (NIH); Ned has lost his mate and is cast out by his friends in the AIDS action group.

These manifest strands of the play seem to us but part of a broader and quite pessimistic vision of human nature and of the world in general that underlies its text, a vision that might explain Kramer's choice of the protest form but also seriously undercuts that form's effectiveness. The audience, the play seems to say, whether gay or straight, is not just separated from AIDS; it is so resistant to hearing about the crisis, and perhaps so thoroughly dulled morally, that only the loudest, most explicit representations will reach it. Only the young, untested Yale students offer any hope of moral or political change.

The embattled isolation of the main characters at the end of *The Normal Heart* is a metaphor for the author's own attitude toward his audience, his belief about our response to the epidemic. On a manifest level, Kramer prods us, but on a deeper level he seems almost to despair of us. This reduced vision of the audience informs a structural pattern in which no "personal" movement occurs that is not also accompanied by "public" content, and it also explains what might be regarded as Kramer's strange choice of someone not suffering from the disease as the main character rather than a person with AIDS himself. Felix's struggle with AIDS is painfully documented in the second half of the play; yet the play's persistent bouts of information and Ned's howls of anger and pain at the imperceptive and uncaring world allow Kramer to hold us at some distance throughout. At the end of the play, all the rest of us, gay or straight, are still found wanting. Only its two heroes are capable of a truly moral stand.

## AS IS

William M. Hoffman's *As Is* is also concerned with the political and social dimensions of AIDS and with "contacting" its audience about the epidemic, but its focus and form are much the reverse of *The Normal Heart*'s and it provides, we believe, a more complete experience of connection for its viewers. In *As Is* the personal and the intimate are at center stage. For instance, we *do* focus here on the world of a person with AIDS; public issues, though not subordinated, are never treated didactically, but are always embodied in dramatic figures and situations. In addition, the play proceeds not in the straight-line manner of *The Normal*

*Heart,* but by a more experimental, "fugal" form that moves both back and forth in time and from foreground to background in the present, a form that demands more from—and thus seems to grant more intelligence to—its audience than do *The Normal Heart*'s linear, literal scenes. Furthermore, and most importantly, given our topic, *As Is* succeeds, we believe, in fully bringing together its characters, its concerns, and its viewers.

In his introduction to the printed version of *As Is*, Hoffman comments on the social and psychic isolation that the sensationalistic and often hostile media treatment of AIDS can enforce on gay men, and he also admits to the anxious desire to distance himself from the disease that he felt as he worked on the play. The key that enabled him to resolve his compositional and psychic problems and to complete the play, he says, was admitting his own fear of contracting AIDS and allowing himself to identify with those who had the disease: "I was willing to go to any lengths for my play, except to imagine myself having AIDS. . . . On a deep irrational level I was terrified of catching it by identifying with those who had it."[3] On every level, *As Is* is concerned with the painful kinds of separation and isolation that AIDS can inflict: the separation of people with AIDS from those without it, whether gay or straight, and the separation of the stigmatized homosexual community, both those with and those without AIDS, from the larger, accepted, heterosexual world. The intention of *As Is*, we believe, is to bring about in its audience, whether homosexual or heterosexual, a version of the kind of identification that Hoffman himself underwent as he wrote the play—to bring gay men closer to their brothers who have AIDS and to bring the supposedly separate and exempt heterosexual audience into closer and more compassionate contact with the world of the play's gay characters.

For the play's gay viewers, the vehicles of that contact would chiefly be the play's gay characters themselves. For the "outsider" heterosexual audience, the vehicles of that contact may most immediately and clearly be characters like the Hospice Worker and the brother of the central figure, Rich. However—and most crucial to the success of *As Is*—the play also contains one recurrent structural element that addresses both of these audiences equally, offering them the common experience of connection to the subject and thus implicitly creating a bridge between them. This is Hoffman's inspired device of the chorus, whose transformations in the course of the play beautifully embody his theme of the need for compassion and contact in the face of the horror and potential divisiveness of AIDS.

*As Is* begins with several different examples of disconnection and isolation. The most evident of these is the first scene between Rich and his former lover, Saul, in which as former live-in lovers attempting a "division of the property," the two men echo the rituals of traditional divorce.

But Hoffman advances this theme in several less obvious ways at the start of the play as well. For instance, the first choral scene, which begins right after Rich announces "I have it" (p. 12), also dramatizes "separating"—here all of the choral figures, homosexual and heterosexual, end by screaming at Rich, "Don't touch me!" (p. 17). One of the most revealing signs of how much this situation of separation and disconnection concerns Hoffman in the play is the way he involves the Hospice Worker in it. It is she whom we meet first in the play, and she is one of the chief figures of identification for the nongay audience. Yet note that she, too, is a "reject" like Rich, for in her opening speech she tells us that after she started working at the AIDS hospice she was expelled from her religious order: Her convent, she says, gave her "the old heave-ho" (p. 3). Opening the play with a character who is not gay and yet is involved in AIDS work is surely one of Hoffman's chief ways of bringing the heterosexual audience closer to the subject or at least of inviting it not to separate immediately from the issue.

The fundamental movement of *As Is* is from these opening instances of separation and disconnection to the final representation of connection and "contact" on every level of the play. These moments of connection occur, most obviously, between the characters—for example, the scene of reconciliation and "forgiveness" between Rich and his brother (pp. 77–81); Saul's later declaration that he will take Rich "as is" (p. 19); and the two men's subsequent "Do you promise?"/"I do" scene between them that echoes a traditional marriage ceremony and that clearly contrasts with the opening "divorce proceedings" between them. The Hospice Worker, too, advances the theme of connection at the end. Though never a "separating" figure, in the speech that closes the play she shows herself to have moved even closer into the supposedly "other" worlds of homosexuality and AIDS as she describes how she painted the fingernails of the dying "queen" "flaming red," dimensionalizing what elsewhere might have simply been a gay male stereotype and providing what in the original New York production was a profoundly moving moment (p. 97).

Hoffman is concerned, however, not just with the achievement of connection between the play's characters, but with affecting connection between the audience and the play's worlds of homosexuality and AIDS as well. It is chiefly through the experimental mode of the choruses of *As Is* (a striking contrast to the journalistic realism of *The Normal Heart*) that Hoffman strives to unite the homosexual and heterosexual members of his audience (for example, by including representatives of each group in them) and to bring both into closer connection with the supposedly "special" worlds on the stage before them. One of the most impressive patterns that emerges from a reading of *As Is* is the transformation that occurs in the content of the play's choruses as the action proceeds, a transformation that subtly recapitulates the movement toward connection that is occurring more obviously on the manifest level of the play. For example, the two choral scenes in the first half of the play are both demonstrations of rejection and separation—the "Don't touch me!" scene already discussed, and the next one, which supplies us with the background of Rich's and Saul's breakup. Then, almost exactly in the middle of the play, as if mirroring the turn from distance to contact that Hoffman is encouraging in his audience throughout, the choral scenes turn from instances of disconnection and selfishness to representations of understanding and compassion. The first choral scene after midpoint is the AIDS support group, where the pregnant heterosexual woman with AIDS says to her fellow members, "You guys know what I mean. You're the only people in the world who know what I mean" (p. 55). And the next is the wonderful hot-line scene with Barney and Pat. Mixing lines like "We're all worried" and "I'm sorry you're lonely" with jibes like "And your mother eats turds in hell" and "If I . . . had it, I'd shove a time bomb up my tush and drop in on Timmy [and] his new lover, Jimmy," and ending with the repetition of "Are you a gay man?"/ "Are you a gay man?" this scene splendidly balances compassion, exasperation, and humor (pp. 60–65).

## CONCLUSION

To have seen *The Normal Heart* and *As Is* in their original New York productions was perhaps chiefly to experience the play's common bonds. But a close reading of the two plays reveals the striking differences in form, focus, and implied audience that we have noted. Just as Kramer's approach could leave his audience with distinctly divided experience—in the way that his approach "contacts" the audience and rejects it at the same time, revealing an underlying pessimism, even despair—Hoffman's form provides as nearly as possible an experience of total "contact" and unity for his audience and implies a correspondingly more optimistic, though never simple minded, world view. The movement in *As Is* from separation to connection on all levels of the play suggests a potential for generosity and moral transformation in the world. Thus, with this complicated fugal form, Hoffman can play with his audience rather than bombard it, and he can give that audience a primary contact with the emotional life of a person with AIDS.

One revealing sign of this spirit of inclusiveness that seems to inform all the levels of *As Is* is the way in which the play handles the issue of promiscuity. *The Normal Heart* leaves its audience with a polar and excluding view of the subject: Once, it seems to say, there was "bad" promiscuity; now there must be "good" chastity. Hoffman, however, while clearly implying that life in the fast lane is over for the gay men who were in it, still tries to bring that bygone mode to his audience's positive attention rather than to banish it. For example, there is an exuberant recitative in which Rich and Saul declare, "God, how I love sleaze . . . Sex. God, I miss it" (pp. 32–35). There is also Saul's "miracle" scene, where, inspired by a vision in front of a Sheridan Square sex shop, he decides against helping Rich commit suicide.

Close scrutiny of *The Normal Heart* and *As Is* can thus alert us as much to the plays' differences as to their similarities and make one of the plays, in our view, a much more profound experience of contact with its subject than the other. Yet both plays still share the common ground we mentioned in starting. As literature, they give concrete, individual form to moral and social issues that in other contexts—ethics books or guides to community organizing—can remain abstract. And as drama they attempt that connection of audience with critical social subject that plays, of all literary forms, can most immediately give.

## NOTES

1. For a survey of these dramas and of other AIDS literature, see D. Altman. *AIDS in the Mind of America*. Garden City, NY: Anchor/Doubleday, 1985, p. 23.

2. L. Kramer. *The Normal Heart*. New York: New American Library, 1985. Citations in the text refer to this edition.

3. W. M. Hoffman. *As Is*. New York: Vintage, 1986, p. xiv. Further page references are to this edition.

# 6 THE AIDS EPIDEMIC: A PHENOMENOLOGICAL ANALYSIS OF THE INFECTIOUS BODY

*Julien S. Murphy*

As the incidence of AIDS rises exponentially, increasing public panic indicates a need to examine the social construction of meanings attached to this disease. A phenomenological analysis of the public's panic response to AIDS shows the influence of pre-existing attitudes toward contagious disease within our cultural stock of knowledge. Specifically, analysis suggests that experience of the AIDS-infected body is structured by a set of phenomenological categories that presuppose both the fear of the body-out-of-control and fear of death. These two fears lie at the root of the social panic over AIDS. A social phenomenological analysis provides a description of how AIDS is experienced in the social world and how the construction of the fear of AIDS casts the epidemic as a modern plague. A reflective response to the AIDS epidemic can show that the difference in meaning between epidemics and plagues is significant for human freedom. Instead of regarding AIDS as a plague, we can wage an authentic revolt against fears and panic, so that we can begin to see how our health forms a primary basis for our interconnectedness with each other and hence forms the basis for human reality.

## AIDS: THE SOCIAL BODY IN DISEASE

As common bearers of a single culture we share a "stock of knowledge" that includes, according to Alfred Schutz, the founder of social phenomenology, assumptions about time, space, the laws of logic, cultural customs, and our own and others' existence. One common assumption that Schutz did not identify is that which I call a "social body." The social body emerges as a central phenomenological concept in an AIDS culture. The social body is not included in the concepts "human species" or "member of the human race." It is not an abstraction from daily life. Rather, it is embedded in our experiences and permeates our awareness of social life. The social body refers to our felt awareness at the prereflective level that the welfare of our own bodies is cogiven with the welfare of others' bodies. The social body gives me my awareness of myself only insofar as I am connected with others both in a collective stream of consciousness and as a body among bodies. *The social body is the lens through which I can differentiate my private body.*

Except in times of plague and epidemic, the social body is a healthy body; we assume that other healthy people both precede and survive us. To the degree that we share health with our contemporaries, we can journey along with others, quietly noting the passing of our lives. It is often the lapse of our own health that brings us not only to a sense of our bodies, but also to the awareness of our death as an immediate possibility. Our bodies are not to be feared as long as health prevails. When our health fails, death, once dim and far away, plunges into our consciousness through the experience of the frailty of our own bodies. Death heightens the fears that accompany our experience of our bodies as contingent grounds for our livelihood.

Fear of the mortality of our bodies is often experienced in bodily nausea. Jean-Paul Sartre described body fear as body nausea even when we are healthy:

A dull and inescapable nausea perpetually reveals my body to my consciousness. Sometimes we look for the pleasant or for physical pain to free ourselves from this nausea; but as soon as the pain and pleasure are *existed by consciousness*, they in turn manifest its facticity and its contingency; and it is on the ground of this nausea that they are revealed. . . . It is on the ground of this nausea that all concrete and empirical nauseas (nausea caused by spoiled meat, fresh blood, excrement, etc.) are produced and make us vomit.[1]

If our experience of our healthy bodies is the foundation for all encounters with nausea, reminding us of our death, then our fears can only be heightened by the unhealthy body in our midst, and most of all the body that suddenly turns ill and cannot be returned to health—the AIDS-infected body.

AIDS reveals the social body in disease.[2] AIDS is present in the "life-world," which Schutz described as "that province of reality which the wide awake . . . adult simply takes for granted in the attitude of common sense."[3] AIDS is far more than a retrovirus, a number of terminally ill people, a death count, or a medical mystery. Whether we think of it or not, AIDS is part of our social experience. AIDS has been built into the layers of the lifeworld, altering our awareness of the social body from one of health to one of fatal disease.

AIDS produces a severe dismemberment of the social body. Not only might we see the body of someone else with AIDS as out of control and near death, but as AIDS continues to spread throughout the country, we begin to fear the entire social body as being out of control and rampant with disease and death. The fear of AIDS becomes manifest in public panic over the fear of the body—the ground of our own mortality. An analysis of the social body in disease requires an examination of how the appearance of AIDS moves into commonsense consciousness, creating body fear and panic in daily social life.

## THE COMMONSENSE AWARENESS OF AIDS

Disease enters the social world on two primary levels: as a *biological event* that infects our bodies and as a *social event* to which a variety of meanings are attached by the choices we make in response to disease. The realization that one has AIDS is the awareness of being infected with a biological and social disease. As the retrovirus infects the physical body of a person, the social virus of AIDS stigmatization enters the net of relationships in which the person lives and works. AIDS becomes a social event, with the constellation of values associated with it highlighting major cultural biases against unconventional sexual behavior and illegal drug use.

Thus, large groups of people become potential patients and are regarded socially as "diseased" simply by being identified as members of high-risk groups: gay or bisexual men, IV drug users, hemophiliacs, sex partners of people with AIDS.

Since AIDS is a highly stigmatized and fatal disease, people at high risk begin watching their bodies for the appearance of the lesions of Kaposi's sarcoma (KS), weight loss, swollen lymph nodes, and insomnia as possible indicators of AIDS. With terror we can find ourselves with AIDS: "I never heard about it [AIDS]," one man says, "until I saw a special on it on 20/20. . . . The special I saw had a man with lesions on it. Mine looked kind of like that, so I went to one of the clinics and they referred me to my doctor. I went to my doctor, and he told me I had AIDS."[4] Another person with AIDS describes a similar process of self-diagnosis common in an epidemic: "I had a series of unexplained blackouts, and eventually when I started hearing what the symptoms of AIDS were, I felt that, you know, I might fit in that category."[5]

People with AIDS describe a sense of disbelief and fear at learning of their diagnosis. "I was told I had cancer, that it was in my blood—systemic—and couldn't be cut out. I was told I probably wouldn't live very long,"[6] recalls one person with AIDS. "I remember a slight sense of disbelief," writes another, "like this wasn't really happening to me."[7]

Many people with AIDS commit their date of diagnosis to memory much like a death sentence. In fact, only 6 percent of all AIDS cases have survived more than three years after diagnosis.[8] Others with, or at high risk for, AIDS commit suicide. Some people with AIDS attempt to reduce the stigma of having the "dreaded disease" by creating a veil of secrecy and telling only a few close friends. Those who choose not to hide their illness are often treated with suspicion by their coworkers, neighbors, and friends. Some people with AIDS are quickly fired from their jobs. Those with AIDS and KS lesions sometimes stay completely out of public view, going out only occasionally to attend a movie, and even then only after the theater lights are out to avoid being seen.

Gay men experience the daily connection between death and sex because thousands of gay men are dying of AIDS, while others see people they have had sex with dying and wonder if AIDS has already been sexually transmitted to them or if future sexual encounters could kill them or their lovers. Young people with or at risk for AIDS experience nearness to death outside of the normal aging cycle. A person with AIDS remarks, "At the age of twenty-eight, I woke up every morning to face the very real possibility of my own death."[9]

Friends, lovers, and relatives of people with AIDS watch near at hand the physical and social effects of the disease on those they love. AIDS accelerates the appearance of the rapid onset of old age; the body degeneration of the elderly appears in formerly healthy gay men aged 20 to 50. One woman writes of her son with AIDS:

Hardest of all was watching a young, healthy man turn into a gaunt, old one, fumbling and shuffling, uncertain and confused. I watched his hair, eyelashes and eyebrows grow sparse and dull. I watched him get so thin that it was too painful to sit on a chair. . . . I lived with his dementia and held him down during his seizures. I never got used to the cane, the wheelchair, the portable commode, and the adult diapers.[10]

The fear of the AIDS-infectious body is found among members of high- and low-risk groups alike. One man noted that worst of all for his old high school friend, a hemophiliac dying of AIDS, was his remorse that he was dying of the "gay disease," that this was the legacy he was leaving to his young son. The friend remarked, "I wanted to hug him. This was the last time I would see him, but several of us were all suited up in gowns and masks and they had me afraid to even touch him."[11] One person with AIDS refers to AIDS patients as being "treated like lepers, who are treated as if they are morally if not literally contagious."[12]

Some gay men shrink from the kiss of greeting, a common practice before AIDS. Others who formerly were quite open about being gay became quiet about it to diminish AIDS fears in others. One gay man remarks, "I have always been out. But I am about to be ordained. If my parish knew I was gay, they would not drink from the same communion cup for fear of catching AIDS."[13] People at low risk re-evaluate their sexual practices in light of AIDS, often afraid of changing relationships for fear that they may increase their exposure to AIDS with a new partner. People buying newspapers, shopping, passing by on city streets begin to notice AIDS media coverage. Some believe that AIDS is just another bad disease, like cancer. Others fear they have already caught it, by chance, or by some rare incident in their past, and become the "worried well," filling AIDS hotlines and doctors' offices, trying to assuage their fears.

The fear that our bodies will be struck with AIDS and become part of the AIDS death count gradually builds into panic. As the panic increases, the possibilities for people with or at high risk for AIDS are severely limited by the worried well. Gay men have not only to deal with the high death rate among lovers and friends but also the spiraling social stigmatization linking AIDS directly to being gay. A gay author writes, "With the onset of AIDS, familiar faces—the man in the bookshop, the mailman, casual acquaintances—began to disappear and funerals became an increasingly frequent part of our lives."[14]

As panic splits the social body between the sick and the healthy, AIDS becomes a plague in commonsense consciousness. Talk of quarantining people with AIDS, or even all persons at high risk, filters through the social world. Some gay establishments are closed down, presumably as a preventive health measure. Hemophiliacs begin experiencing suspicion at the workplace. Some children with AIDS are banned from school. One gay man learning of a friend who came down with pneumocystis pneumonia, a symptom of AIDS, recalls, "Another friend rushed up weeping with a copy of *New York Magazine* and said, this is what he's got. The article was entitled 'The Gay Plague,' and it was so hysterical that pretty soon we were hysterical ourselves."[15] A reviewer of a recent gay film comments, "This is the post-gay liberation world of New York, in the plague years of the 80's."[16]

## IS AIDS "THE MODERN PLAGUE?"

There has never been an illness like it in modern times. AIDS stands today as the most serious and threatening medical and social phenomenon—the single greatest public health menace—of the age.

*The Boston Globe*

The metaphor of AIDS as plague has quietly slipped into common-sense ways of thinking about the disease. The media in particular have spread the myth of AIDS as plague, the "gay plague," with headlines such as "Gay Plague Baffling Medical Detectives" and "Gay Plague Has Arrived in Canada."[17] Even a recent public policy conference was entitled "AIDS: A Modern Plague?"[18] Undoubtedly, AIDS is "the greatest public health crisis in the twentieth century" and perhaps even "the most virulent epidemic known to man."[19] Nonetheless, it is vital to the freedom of us all that this epidemic not be seen as a plaguelike phenomenon, for such a metaphorical shift only heightens the oppressive stigmatization of people with or at risk for AIDS.

Unlike the word "epidemic," "plague" creates a mystique of moral blame around the plague-stricken. The figurative meanings of plague refer to a scourge, an evil, an act of divine anger, divine punishment. Plague can mean disease serving a moral purpose, namely, to cleanse the world of undesirables, such as the ten plagues of Egypt. Since the AIDS-afflicted are already judged to be socially undesirable, the plague metaphor for AIDS can only increase negative judgments about people with AIDS and suggest that AIDS is an instance of divine punishment. If AIDS is seen as plague, a further ostracism of all high-risk persons will result. It is possible that everything associated with a high-risk person could be seen as "infected," leading to a severing of the social body between the clean and the allegedly impure.

The host of plague-related words that have been used in the past, such as "plague bill," "plague house," "plague pit," "plague mark," "plague water," "plague cake," "plaguer," "plaguey," evidence how easily superstitions can reach into and transform daily social life.

AIDS, like plague, does appear by surprise, is incurable, and does bring disease and death. But AIDS need not disrupt the social order, our set of beliefs about life, or our relationships to each other. AIDS is, after all, a sexually transmitted disease as well as a disease spread by contaminated needles or blood products. Current medical research reports that AIDS is not spread by casual contact. Hence, whereas it may have been appropriate to fear interacting with people during the bubonic plague, no medical evidence exists to support the fear that we can "catch" AIDS from each other, short of engaging in unsafe sexual practices or sharing infected blood or needles. All of us can, to a large extent, protect ourselves from AIDS. Very sound and effective precautions can be taken against AIDS that are not based on fear or superstition and that need not be oppressive, namely, education and accessibility to safe sex materials, legalization of the distribution of sterile needles to drug users, and routine screening of blood donations. Yet despite sound precautions, many people persist in believing that it may be possible to catch AIDS from casual contact, and have an irrational distrust of any medical claims about AIDS. They thus project their own fears onto a retrovirus they perceive as entirely uncontrollable.

People acting against the prevalent medical opinion of the time collectively create hysteria, which culminates in news stories of bizarre ways AIDS may be transmitted, beyond people's control. People are warned that "No American Is Safe"; "If you live in a neighborhood in New York City with a high level of mosquitoes, you may well be at risk [for AIDS]";[20] and even that "AIDS may be passed thru Laundry [sic]."[21] Such irrational fears are unproductive and maintain the oppression of people with AIDS.

The irrational fear of AIDS in "plague" thinking suggests that AIDS may be, in commonsense consciousness, the disease of the nuclear age. AIDS brings to the individual, like the nuclear threat that looms over our culture, the imminent threat of total annihilation. The AIDS retrovirus can suddenly appear in one's body as if coming from nowhere, and by the time it appears, it is too late for the body to defend itself, even against otherwise nonfatal opportunistic infections. Moreover, we find paralleling the AIDS epidemic, a highly infeasible military strategy. The Strategic Defense Initiative can be seen as a reaction to AIDS. At a time when members of our culture are dying in great numbers from a retrovirus that immobilizes their own bodies' immune system, a perfect immune system is projected onto outer space in our country's military strategies—a nuclear shield so powerful that President Reagan describes it, in the early period of the AIDS epidemic (1983), as ultimately enabling us to "intercept and destroy strategic ballistic missiles before they [reach] our own soil or that of our allies."[22] Both the AIDS epidemic and the Strategic Defense Initiative reflect a specific fear that accompanies the fears of death and of the body-out-of-control—the fear of total vulnerability. The largest threats to total vulnerability are AIDS and nuclear war. Despite our technology, which enables us to control many events, we are still vulnerable to disease and death.

It is possible to curb the hysteria and fear about AIDS not by denying our fear of total vulnerability but by waging an authentic resistance to AIDS at the existential level through a philosophy of revolt. A philosophy of revolt against AIDS acknowledges the social body as the vital network of our interconnections to each other and emphasizes human freedom as the highest goal for a social community.

## AIDS AND REVOLT

From now on it can be said that plague was the concern of all of us. Hitherto, each individual citizen had gone about his business as usual, and no doubt he would have continued. But once the gates were shut, once we were all in the same boat, each would have to adapt himself to the new conditions of life—the ache of separation and the fear was shared alike.[23]

A philosophy of existential revolt is found in Albert Camus's novel, *The Plague*, in which a town infested with bubonic plague is used to depict a social community with a social illness: fascism. Camus portrays an existential philosophy of revolt by stressing that, at the core of the human condition, both freedom and goodness link us in vital connection to each other. He suggests a dichotomy in the social world between those who choose to be pestilences and those who are the victims of pestilence, and calls for a path of healing and peace that enables us to mount an authentic revolt against all forms of oppression and even to revolt against death itself.

Camus claims that we are free to shape the values of the social world. We are responsible for our own destinies and for the level of social oppression, or social infection, in the social body: "What's natural is the microbe. All the rest—health, integrity, purity (if you like)—is a product of the human will, a vigilance that must never falter."[24] Camus is aware that the creation of oppressive values, such as the stigmatizing of people with or at high risk for AIDS, is always possible because we are the makers and sustainers of human values. Yet his novel refuses an attitude of wariness toward human beings and suggests instead a rugged hopefulness in the goodness of others. At the same time that he warns we are free to choose tyranny ("the plague bacillus never dies or disappears for good, . . . it can lie dormant for years, . . ."[25]) the narrator of the novel affirms that the lesson of plague is insight into human goodness. Dr. Rieux writes: "What we learn in time of pestilence: that there are more things to admire in men than to despise."[26]

An existential philosophy of revolt resists oppressive values that stigmatize people with and at high risk for AIDS by refusing to cast judgment on people needlessly. For Camus, there are no absolute values save a hope for goodness and freedom. We each must choose our paths in life for ourselves and on our own terms. Similarly, there is no deep meaning to life itself, except for the meanings we create. There is no deep message in getting AIDS. No one deserves to have AIDS. Each of us has before us the constant task of giving our lives meaning, even though much of what happens to us may be beyond our control, or absurd. Through the character of Tarrou in *The Plague*, Camus emphasizes the tyranny of choosing to judge others when their actions commit no harm. Such judgment is to pass a death sentence on others, to bring death into the social world by limiting the freedom of others needlessly:

> All I maintain is that on this earth there are pestilences and there are victims, and it's up to us, so far as possible, not to join forces with the pestilences. . . . I grant . . . a third category: that of the true

healers. But it's a fact one doesn't come across many of them . . . and anyhow it must be a hard vocation. That's why I decided to take, in every predicament, the victim's side, so as to reduce the damage done. Among them I can at least try to discover how one attains to the third category; in other words, to peace.[27]

Tarrou believes that everyone has plague, that we all risk infecting each other at the level of human freedom and possibilities. But through Tarrou, Camus suggests that we can be vigilant about the values we bring into and maintain in the social world, that we can strive to reduce the damage done in respect to the lived situation of AIDS, and that, moreover, we can attempt to be healers of the social body in the midst of an epidemic instead of spreading harm.

An existential philosophy of revolt against AIDS recognizes the ambiguity of choices amidst risk factors for our physical and social health. Whereas epidemiologists define the level of biological risk for AIDS, existentialists continually evaluate the risks for freedom we take by our social activities in regard to AIDS. It is our task to measure, with a gambler's eye, our own balance between risk and safety. Whether a high-risk individual practices safe sex or not, whether an IV drug user chooses safe needle use, whether a person with AIDS decides to accept or refuse medical care or gives in to despair or revolt, whether all of us choose to spread the plague myth about AIDS or fight against it, and to what degree, are in the end the measures of our own value. As Camus writes, each of our lives, particularly evident in epidemic, "could be only the record of what had to be done, and what assuredly would have to be done again in the never ending fight against terror and its relentless onslaughts, despite their personal afflictions, by all who, unable to be saints but refusing to bow down to pestilences, strive their utmost to be healers."[28]

An existential revolt against AIDS, like any authentic striving for meaning, is also a revolt against death. It is absurd that we all die, if not of AIDS, then of something else. Although we cannot choose not to die, we can choose, within our own situations, the risks we will take with others, and with our health, in ways that help us live ever more deeply. In some respects, AIDS is yet another instance of our mortality. AIDS brings us to a confrontation of the absurdity of death and the desire to make life meaningful. Camus suggests that the creation of meaning always happens within the frame of life and death. Reflecting on the death of Tarrou from plague, Dr. Rieux concludes that what we really have in life is knowledge of friendship and its memories and that, sifting through all of our experiences of ourselves and others, what we can retain is the limits of our knowledge: "Knowing meant that: a living warmth and a picture of death."[29] Within the framework of living warmth and an image of death, we take up our lives, choosing either revolt or despair, resistance to oppression or fear.

A phenomenological analysis of the AIDS-infectious body reveals two general responses to the biological and social threats of AIDS: a panic arising from fear of death and the body-out-of-control and an existential revolt against the social oppression of having AIDS. The former response can only lead to irrational consequences that may jeopardize the rights of persons with or at high risk for AIDS, specifically the rights to freedom, adequate health care, and social possibilities. The latter response offers to maintain our essential freedom and stresses our interconnections with each other as members of a social body in which the value of each of us is linked to the values all of us create. It thus encourages sound social policy on AIDS issues. Such a philosophy of revolt against AIDS can define and evaluate the dilemmas of choice and risk inherent not only in epidemics of contagious disease, such as AIDS, but in the health of social life altogether.

## NOTES

1. J. P. Sartre. *Being and Nothingness*; trans. H. E. Barnes. New York: Washington Square Press, 1953, p. 445.

2. This analysis specifically addresses the lived experience of AIDS in the United States. Also, much of what is said about AIDS applies to AIDS-related complex (ARC).

3. A. Schutz and T. Luckmann. *The Structures of the Lifeworld*, trans. R. M. Zaner and T. H. Engelhardt, Jr. Evanston, IL: Northwestern University Press, 1973, p. 3.

4. G. L. Nungesser. Interview with Lance Gaines. *Epidemic of Courage: Facing AIDS in America*. New York: St. Martin's Press, 1986, p. 53.

5. Ibid., interview with Bob Cecchi, 25.

6. Ibid., interview with Dan Turner, 90–91.

7. Nungasser, *Epidemic of Courage*, 48.

8. *New York Times* (June 16, 1986):B10, C5. As of June 9, 11,731 of the 21,517 total cases of AIDS reported to the Centers for Disease Control in Atlanta had died.

9. D. Altman. *AIDS in the Mind of America*. New York: Anchor/Doubleday, 1986, p. 6; from a speech by Michael Callen to the New York congressional delegation, May 10, 1983.

10. B. Peabody. A family faces AIDS with love. Portland, ME. *Our Paper* (August 1985).

11. Research for this paper included phenomenological interviews with people with or at high risk for AIDS, students and staff of the Harvard Festival of Life, and staff of the Fenway Community Health Center and AIDS Action Committee, Boston, February 1986.

12. Altman, *AIDS*, 6.

13. Interviews.

14. Altman, *AIDS*, 1.

15. Nungesser, *Epidemic of Courage*, interview with Armistead Maupin, 206.

16. D. Ansen. When being gay is a fact of life. *Newsweek* (June 9, 1986):80.

17. Altman, *AIDS*, 17.

18. Conference, AIDS: A Modern Plague? The Medical, Legal, Ethical and Public Policy Issues. Boston, MA, April 3–5, 1986.

19. F. P. Siegal and M. Siegal. *AIDS: The Medical Mystery*. New York: Grove Press, 1983, coverflap text quoted from *Newsweek*; P. A. Giudici and W. A. Check. *The Truth about AIDS: Evolution of an Epidemic*. New York: Holt Rinehart Winston, 1984, coverflap text.

20. Cover story. *Weekly World News* (March 25, 1986):1.

21. AIDS may be passed thru laundry. *Sun* (June 17, 1986):25.

22. R. Reagan. Address to the nation on defense and national security, March 23, 1983. *Public Papers of the President of United States: Ronald Reagan, 1983*. Washington, D.C.: U.S. Government Printing Office, 1984, p. 442.

23. A. Camus. *The Plague*. New York: Vintage Books, 1972, p. 63.

24. Ibid.

25. Ibid., 287.

26. Ibid.

27. Ibid., 236.

28. Ibid., 287.

29. Ibid., 271.

# II The Clinical Experience of AIDS

# 7 DUTIES, FEARS, AND PHYSICIANS
*Erich H. Loewy*

Two events inclined me to think about the issue of a physician's duty in the face of fears. Both involved physician refusal to care for an AIDS patient—the one involved a surgeon refusing to operate, the other a pathologist refusing to autopsy such a patient. They pleaded fear of contagion, and in both cases the response of peers and community was ambivalent. No one really wished to confront this issue at a more than technical level. As one who deals a great deal with ethics—or at least one who talks a lot about it—I was troubled. A search of the literature dealing with this problem, whether the specific or the generic one, yielded almost no fruit and a search of my own and my colleagues' souls left me equally perplexed. Believing the issue to be far more important and far-reaching than these specific instances, I decided to explore it and to share some of my thoughts and concerns.

## DUTY, FEAR, AND COURAGE IN THE MEDICAL SETTING

This chapter deals with the relationship of physicians to some of their fears, the nature of those fears, and the physician's duty in response to them. For the current purpose, I shall define fear as a sensation or a feeling of anxiety caused by a realization, perception, or expectation of impotency in the face of perceived or expected danger or evil. It sub-

Reprinted with permission from *Social Science and Medicine* 22, Erich H. Loewy, "Duties, Fears, and Physicians," Copyright © 1986, Pergamon Journals Ltd.

sumes such qualities as dread and awe, and as will be seen later, other emotive and aesthetic elements enter into it. Duty will be defined as an obligation assumed by moral agents in recognition of the moral law as distilled through their society. Courage—another necessary element in this discussion—is defined as the "disposition to voluntarily act, perhaps fearfully, in a dangerous circumstance . . . "; its "essence is the mastery of fear for the preservation of a perceived good against dangers." Courage is an important element in our discussion because courage makes possible action consonant with duty in the face of fear. Duty, fear, and courage are inextricably linked in the analysis of the physician's role.[1]

Physicians as a group reflect the society from which they arise and in which they serve. The relationship is reciprocal and mutually sustaining. Attitudes and values of a society are, to some extent, shared by any group within it, and those attributes and values in turn are influenced by the nature of the experiences peculiar to the group. The group shares the fears and values of its society. These values and fears are not special or different in kind but rather are abstracted from those prevalent in the community. Persons who incline toward medicine as a profession often have a somewhat different hierarchy of values and fears. Experience further modifies these, lessening some and accentuating others. Medicine's role within a community produces a unique complexion of expectations in the community which, in turn, is reflected in the physician's perception of duty.

There are, of course, many elements that enter into the concept "fears." Repugnance adds to fear and with fear may preclude action. We may fear to be shocked by some apparatus at the bedside but may overcome this fear and, if need be, manipulate it. Yet, when the same instrument is covered with slime, we may not do so. The two sensations—disgust and fear in this case—are mutually reinforcing and preclude action. Physicians fearing contagion unassociated with other repulsive qualities may—with fear and trembling, perhaps—treat the patient. But if, in addition, the disease is associated in their minds with strong negative aesthetic or moral considerations, they may fail to act. In many people's minds AIDS carries a *connotation* of sin, a remnant of the belief in disease as "God's punishment," and this produces revulsion in the physician. Together with the fear of contagion such feelings may preclude action.

In dealing with the role of the physician's fear vis-à-vis duty, it is necessary to recognize clearly that fear does not always oppose duty. Fear of censure, fear of losing prestige and, perhaps most important of all, fear of losing one's own self-esteem may act as powerful forces. There is the fear of acting and the fear of shirking one's duty. Fear here opposes fear. Both discharging and not discharging one's duty now takes courage.

## HISTORICAL CONSIDERATIONS

Have physicians throughout history had the assumed obligation to treat patients despite personal risk? Before using epidemic disease as a paradigm for this examination, we must be sure that the society examined recognized epidemics in the light of contagion through personal contact rather than as an affliction unrelated to this. There is sound evidence that this was the case during most of the principle "plagues." In describing the plague of Athens (fifth century B.C.) Thucydides mentions the disproportionate number of physicians who died taking care of patients.[2] Hippocrates [460–370 B.C.] gives physicians careful instructions for the purification of the air. He implied that physicians must stay, help the patient, and guard themselves against infection as well as they could. This, although until about the sixteenth century physicians were not expected to treat the irreversibly sick—a tradition counter to our current beliefs and dating back to pre-Hippocratic times.[3] Galen in the second century of our era fled Rome during the Antonine plague despite his fears that he would be brought back in chains by an angry Marcus Aurelius whose physician he was. He found it necessary to develop an elaborate series of excuses and apologies for his actions, and the attempt to excuse him continues to this day.[4]

During the Justinian plague—which undoubtedly was what we call plague today (that is, caused by *Yersinia pestis*)[5] and which lasted from about A.D. 540 to 590—both pneumonic and bubonic forms ravaged the Western world. Procopius[6] not only gives us a superb description of the times, its social mechanism, and its history, but also gives us an excellent clinical description of the disease. He speaks of "physicians examining the bodies of the dead" and of the function of physicians during those times. It is evident that the internal life of Byzantium continued without severe internal disruption—albeit with the gravest consequences for Justinian's self-imposed mission of creating a Byzantine Roman Empire.[7] Had physicians deserted, severe disruption could hardly have been avoided. From primitive times to the present, communities have needed their healers to feel secure.

The Black Death that coursed through Europe from 1348 to 1350 killed between one-third and one-half of the population, and repetitive pulses of plague intermittently scourged Europe until the seventeenth century.[8] These plagues, and especially those in the fourteenth century, form an excellent example of social response to epidemic disease.[9] There is a relative wealth of historical and literary material available for this period.[10] The contagious nature of the disease was well understood, even if the mechanism of contagion was not. The entire public—from the Pope sweating between two huge fires in Avignon to the serf desperate in his thatched hut—was well aware of this. Children deserted parents, husbands and wives deserted each other, and even young children were abandoned by their parents—so desperate was the fear of contagion. Society was maddened.[11] Troops of flagellants roamed the streets, scourging each other and killing the Jews.[12] Prayer vigils alternated with or encompassed riotous orgies,[13] and increasingly hunger stalked the streets as crops were left untended and cattle died. But societal dislocation may not have been as complete as once thought. Magistrates largely continued to perform their duties, and when they died, others took their place; wills were written and probated; priests gave last rites; physicians made their appointed rounds.[14] The social contract—implicit but reinforced by fear of censure—held. Not always, not everywhere, and not for everyone— but enough so that the sorely wrinkled fabric of society was not completely torn asunder. When it was all over, structure rather than anarchy resulted. The magistrates, the priests, the physicians—many ran but apparently many more stayed, died, and in dying preserved moral continuity between their age and to us.[15] Why did they stay? Perhaps they shared the view of Guy de Chauliac:" . . . and I, to avoid infamy, dared not absent myself but with continual fear preserved myself as best I could. . . . "[16] De Chauliac contracted plague, survived, and continued to care for its victims. His statement shows the agony of being torn by conflicting fears and conflicting perceptions of duty. In Perugia, Gentile da Foligno methodically autopsied victims, enriched our knowledge, and fell prey to the plague. Those who did not stay were held in contempt both in reality and in the mirror that fiction holds up to society. The doctrine, violated to be sure by some but honored by most, held—a physician does not desert his patients.[17]

From the period of the Black Death until the late seventeenth or eighteenth century, sporadic epidemics of plague racked parts of Europe. During this time, a few municipalities appointed specific "pest-doctors," contractually obliged to remain during epidemics, and others passed laws forbidding physicians to leave during epidemics. But most did not. Such physicians were the forerunners of our public health officials, and they served a similar function. The exceptional physician left his patients; most stayed. During London's "Great Plague" in the summer of 1665[18] a meeting of the Royal College was adjourned because plague "rages much about the town." Sydenham and a few others fled but many more, like Glisson and Wharton, stayed.[19] In the yellow fever epidemics of the eighteenth century in Philadelphia some physicians fled but many more, among them Benjamin Rush, stood their ground. In even more modern times, physicians did not flee during the great pandemic that followed World War I. They stayed and worked, and many died. Later, during the severe polio epidemics, in infectious disease hospitals and in sanatoriums, physicians unquestioningly (or questioningly) assumed risks. I shall not belabor the point. Throughout history society expected its functionaries to continue their duties in good times and in bad.[20] It gave them considerable benefits—material as well as those derived from status, prestige, and power. In return, it expected from them behavior bespeaking a sense of duty and honor. Some violated the contract; many more, it seems, did not. Praise for those who stayed was more muted than was the definite censure for those who fled. "To avoid infamy"—that speaks volumes in this regard and it has continued to speak to us down through the ages.

## A VIEW OF THE SOCIAL CONTRACT AND THE PROFESSION

Our view of the physician's duty in the face of the fear of "coming to harm" is implicitly grounded in our view of the social contract. This tacit understanding among the members of a community underpins and has always underpinned the community's functioning. While this understanding may seem to limit freedom—and to some extent it certainly does—it allows society to function and thereby maximizes freedom for all. Without this tacit understanding—enforced here and there by law[21]— disruption would occur and functioning could continue only by coercion of the weak by the strong. Enforcement of this contract is frequently through social mechanisms involving praise, centure, and even stigmatization, with all its consequences for the individual. That contract does not always operate smoothly; it is often ignored. The affluent industrialist in ignoring social conditions, the wealthy nation glutted with food amidst world hunger ignore the contract to their ultimate peril. But here the relationships are not one to one, are even more complicated; therefore, the consequences, while more severe, are longer in coming. For while the larger contract may be violated, its one-to-one dimension is upheld. The individual person who is a member and product of that society is more immediately involved in and responsive to the contract on a one-to-one basis.

A social contract does not resolve fear but it necessitates dealing with fear so that appropriate action results. Within the confines of the contract there is the understanding that action—even if not feelings—will be congruous with the contract. Without this the contract is meaningless. No specific contract is for life, for we are not the same person throughout our existence, even though a broad identity persists. But as long as the contract is in force, as long as it has not been abrogated—and abrogated publicly and ostensively—it must be observed.

Physicians can abrogate their contract just as can other members of the community. Logically, this can only be done when the situation is not acute and when, therefore, such abrogation does not rip the social fabric. Physicians can abrogate the contract by leaving the profession or narrow it by limiting their field of practice. But however done, it must be done publicly and with due notice. For example, a pathologist cannot selectively refuse to autopsy the victims of contagion unless at some time prior to the occasion such an understanding has been reached. Internists can refuse to care for the syphilitic or the leprous only if they have publicly stated this exclusion and have been heard by their community; the limitation is of the same order as any other accepted limitation or condition of their practice. It holds under "ordinary" circumstances. But even when limitation has occurred, circumstances may alter it—an internist (not ordinarily expected to deliver babies) is expected to deliver a baby when isolated from other medical help and an obstetrician may be expected to treat a heart attack victim under similar conditions. That is implicitly understood within that broader contract, and violations inevitably result in censure, stigma and, in some parts of the world, in legal action. The professional, having made a commitment, remains bound by it. The degree of that bond varies with the situation encountered but some bond remains.

The meaning of being a professional in medicine, according to Pellegrino,[22] is that the doctor has "professed to perform a good act of healing when confronted with the fact of illness." He or she has professed expertise in the appropriate field and has tacitly or explicitly professed a willingness to exercise this expertise. Willingness, then, makes the expertise operative. When a professional is licensed or given a degree, willingness is presumed in testing for expertise. Its exercise relies on an implicit social contract. Willingness to perform a technically "good" act necessarily involves choices—choices of what is "good" and what is "bad," choices that involve technical options as means and often suggest ends committed to ethical values. The choice made, then, is a decision based upon a composite of fact and value. And these facts, too, in a more tacit and less conscious way, are underpinned by values. For facts do not come to us naked and complete; they are endowed with and chosen through the slowly developing values of a lifetime. And among the many factors underlying the choice are emotive ones—ones that deal with hope as well as with fear.

What does "to be willing" mean? Willingness to proceed with a task implies the realization that some negative element—obstacles, fear, or pain—may be connected with the task. To be willing to do a given thing that is totally without perceived negative elements is almost tautologous. The assumption of risk, then, is an implicit element of "being willing." To be a will, the will must potentially be disposed to pit itself against trouble in the discharge of its task. Will implies choice, determination, and purpose. The task before us may be almost entirely pleasant, but in expressing a willingness for the undertaking negative elements have been assumed. To be willing to choose a life's work is to be ready to assume negative factors as a by-product of what is perceived as desirable. It may be the case that advantages fail to materialize and that, instead, unrealized unpleasantness and even unanticipated dangers present themselves. And if that is the case, it is plausible to "change one's mind" either by abandoning or by altering some aspects of the profession. But that can only be done (and be moral) with due notice before a task is in sight and not, as it were, after the task has presented itself. Professional integrity demands the fulfillment of a person's social contract. Without this, the profession of skill is empty.

## A VIEWPOINT OF OBLIGATION

Many factors enter into our clinical and personal decisions. A "decision" is a composite and its expression is an "action"—be it the "doing of something" or the "not doing" of that thing. Before a decision is reached, technical options outlining the realm of the possible must be ascertained. These provide answers to such questions as what kind of risk? how much risk? and is protection possible and available? The answers here are crucial to our moral consideration. If undertaking a given course would result in certain death, a different set of considerations pertains than if the risk is small. And even in the first instance, there is a critical difference between the act of giving one's life to save another and giving one's life without any chance of saving that other. Risks also differ in terms of how we "come to harm"—harm in terms of life, pain, material loss, or separation.

Physicians are not asked to assume a risk of certain death or infection. In the past, they were expected to assume reasonable risks—reasonable within the context of their community and of the situation there. Only rarely did this expectation find contractual or legal expression. There were a few municipalities that bound certain physicians to service, such as the "pestdoctors-physicians." There were a few that threatened legal reprisal in case of desertion. But there were only a few. Most relied on the much weightier stricture of conscience induced by the tacit social contract. In those times, furthermore, some of the "fleeing" was debatable—the Sydenhams treated mainly upper-class patients. These often fled and, in a sense, Sydenham fled *with* rather than *from* his patients. And still, there was evident guilt as expressed by the need to explain and defend. Today, this is not the case. Our patients are among us and epidemics rage, chronicled daily in the media. The danger of death or of serious harm to us through our administrations—while not entirely known—is fairly well understood and hardly formidable. Physicians faced greater risk in treating infection before antimicrobials were available and did not shrink from that risk. What underlies our fears, what has changed our sense of duty?

Explanations abound. No longer is the society in which physicians are rooted and in which they function the "tight little island" of yesteryear. In many respects it is more egocentric, more hedonistic, more pampered and spoiled, less community oriented, and more dedicated to the self. Individuals have lower moral expectations for themselves but often have raised them for others. Our media and our propaganda extol "rugged individualism" and often demean social action. Running risks for purposes of social benefit does not sit well with us. We physicians have been spoiled. We are used to curing formerly fatal infections. Infectious disease not subject to cure elicits an unaccustomed fear and challenges our God-like invincibility. It brings us face to face with the fact that we are finite and mortal, and we do not like it.[23]

AIDS is subtly different in another way as well. It is seen as a category of "venereal" disease even if, as with other such diseases, its transmission is not exclusively venereal. There is sham moral repugnance with a special wrinkle—it is "venereal" under especially repugnant circumstances. There is the tacit but very real flavor of sin and God's just punishment. Often these feelings add to the primary fear of contagion and induce physicians to violate their social contract.

I have tried to show that an enduring social contract binds healers to their community. The contract has endured through the ages and in many cultures. Both physician and community have profited—the physician has been blessed with immense privileges, prerogatives, and power as well as with considerable material reward; the community, which has profited from the healer's skills, assumes that the contract will be honored in time of need. If medicine honors its contract, medicine in turn is deserving of honor; if the contract is broken, medicine will be deserving of the infamy that De Chauliac feared.

## NOTES

1. E. E. Shelp. Courage: A neglected virtue in the patient-physician relationship. *Social Science and Medicine* 18 (1984):351–60.

2. A. Jonsen. Personal communication.

3. D. W. Amundsen. The physician's obligation to prolong life: A medical duty without classical roots. *Hastings Center Report* 8 (August 1978):23–31.

4. J. Walsh. Refutation of the charges of cowardice against Galen. *Annals of Medical History* 3 (1931):195–208.

5. T. L. Bratton. The identity of the plague of Justinian. *Transactions and Studies of the College of Physicians of Philadelphia* 3 (1981):113–24, 174–80. C. Russell. That earlier plague. *Demography* 5 (1968):179–84.

6. Procopius. *History of the Wars; Secret History; Buildings.* New Haven, CT: Twayne, 1967.

7. A. Cameron. *Continuity and Change in Sixth-Century Byzantium.* London: Variorum Reprints, 1981.

8. H. E. Sigerist. *Civilization and Disease*. Chicago: University of Chicago Press, 1943.

9. G. Marks. *The Medieval Plague*. New York: Doubleday, 1971.

10. G. Boccaccio. *The Decameron*. New York: New American Library, 1982. C. M. Cipolla. *Cristofano and the Plague*. Los Angeles: University of California Press, 1973. W. Bullein. *A Dialogue Against the Fever Pestilence*. Oxford: Oxford University Press, 1931. First published 1888.

11. W. L. Langer. The black death. *Scientific American* 210 (1961):114–21.

12. J. Nohl. *The Black Death*. San Francisco: Harper & Bros., 1924 and see Marks, *Medieval Plague*.

13. A. Deux. *The Black Death, 1347*. London: Weybright-Tolley, 1969.

14. E. W. Emery. The black death of 1348 in Perpignan. *Speculum* 42 (1967):511–623.

15. D. William, ed. *The Black Death: The Impact of the 14th Century Plague*. Binghamton, NY: Medieval & Renaissance Texts and Studies, SUNY-Binghamton, 1982.

16. A. M. Campbell. *The Black Death and Men of Learning*. New York: AMS Press, 1966.

17. D. W. Amundsen. Medical deontology and the pestilential diseases in the late middle ages. *Journal of the History of Medicine and Allied Sciences* 32 (1977):403–21.

18. D. Defoe. *A Journal of the Plague Year*. Oxford: Basil-Blackwell, 1928.

19. I. Veith. Medical ethics through the ages. *Annual Bulletin of Northwestern University Medical School* 31 (1957):351–58.

20. G. Rath. Arztliche ethik in pestzeiten. *Munchener Medizinische Wochenschrift* 99 (1957):158–62.

21. S. D'Irsay. Defense reactions during the black death, 1348–1349. *Annals of Medical History* 9 (1927):169–79.

22. E. D. Pellegrino. Toward a reconstruction of medical morality: The primacy of the act of profession and the fact of illness. *Journal of Medicine and Philosophy* 4 (1979):32–55.

23. E. H. Loewy. AIDS and the physician's duty to treat (editorial). *Chest* 89 (1986):325–26.

# 8 PHYSICIAN RESPONSE TO A NEW, LETHAL, AND PRESUMABLY INFECTIOUS DISEASE: MEDICAL RESIDENTS AND THE AIDS EPIDEMIC IN SAN FRANCISCO

*Barbara A. Koenig and Molly Cooke*

The AIDS epidemic—patients dying of a lethal, infectious disease. It is already difficult to recall a time when this deadly illness was not constantly in the public mind. And fear. We have probably all experienced it to some degree. But what of physicians? Are they immune? One author has suggested that physicians have responded with "an atavistic terror" to the "ancient fear of contagion."[1] How have healers reacted to AIDS? And in particular, how did medical residents in San Francisco, an early focus of the epidemic, respond? Although the answers to these questions are enormously complicated, informed by personal courage, strength, and occasional prejudice, the response to AIDS reveals much about the basic tensions at the heart of modern medicine. The medical residency, one of the most difficult and stressful times in a physician's career, is not simply a period during which one learns technical skills. It is also a moral apprenticeship, during which the novice physician learns at first hand the nature of medical responsibility. This includes the paradox of two seemingly opposed sets of duties: one to patients, the other, usually less well articulated, to self. AIDS tells us much about this conflict.

## STUDY DESIGN AND METHODS

This chapter presents the results of a study of physician response to the AIDS epidemic. Patients, of course, bear the main burden of AIDS. But as the epidemic unfolded we became aware that AIDS was having a major impact on residents in the internal medicine training program at the University of California at San Francisco (UCSF). Our study, conducted in 1983, used a combination of two research strategies: questionnaires plus intensive interviewing.

Residents in the UCSF training program in internal medicine were the study population. Methods included an anonymous pencil-and-paper questionnaire given to all residents in the program. Sixty residents returned questionnaires, a response rate of 54 percent. It was hoped that the anonymous format would allow residents to express freely their feelings about the AIDS epidemic. In addition to the questionnaire, an interview study was conducted of members of one cohort in the training program.[2] Thirty-three second-year residents—94 percent of the total— were interviewed in the period immediately following completion of their internship on the wards of the three UCSF teaching hospitals. Their internship year (the period of residency training in which physicians have the most intense contact with patients) coincided with a geometric increase in the number of AIDS patients and the first public awareness of the extent of the AIDS problem.

The interview study was part of a large anthropological study of house officer training in the care of dying patients.[3] The questions asked in the interviews were completely open-ended, designed to elicit the resident's response to the AIDS epidemic as a whole. We feel that the two methods (open-ended interviews and a forced-choice questionnaire) complement each other, one allowing a demographic and quantitative assessment of the response to AIDS and the other allowing insight into the nature of resident response to AIDS.

## CONTEXT

Before discussing the study results it is essential to review the social and medical context of the study period. Data collection took place in the summer and early fall of 1983, relatively early in the epidemic. AIDS did not become a household word overnight. Rather, the national concern which we now take for granted took time to develop. A key fact to keep in mind is that at the time of this study, scientific acceptance of the isolation of the virus presumed to cause AIDS had not occurred. Although Luc Montagnier announced the discovery of an "AIDS virus" in April, 1983, the idea that a particular retrovirus causes AIDS was not generally accepted until Gallo's announcement in May 1984.[4] Certainly most medical personnel worked under the assumption that AIDS was caused by a virus with transmission patterns similar to hepatitis B. But it is important to keep in mind that the exact cause of AIDS remained unknown during the study period. Similarly, the degree of risk to health workers caring for AIDS patients, although now known to be quite low,[5] was not known with certainty.

Documenting a climate of fear is difficult but necessary because physicians are not immune to generalized public reactions. One indication of the public "climate of opinion" with regard to AIDS is the media attention devoted to the disease. The number of articles about AIDS in local newspapers increased suddenly in the early summer of 1983. During those months stories appeared almost daily, whereas previously there were few articles, ranging from none to eight per month. The first peak of public concern was in June 1983, when the *San Francisco Examiner* published 44 AIDS articles.[6] The increased media coverage of AIDS coincided with the first reports of transfusion-related cases, changing the locus of concern for the disease from a small and socially stigmatized minority to the general "blameless" population. Our study took place shortly after the first dramatic increase in public concern about the disease.

Although public concern began to peak in June 1983, we believe that physician concern about AIDS actually peaked earlier. Our observations of the training program suggest that the peak concern for general physicians and residents in the UCSF medicine training program occurred six months earlier, in about December 1982 or January 1983. It was at this time that a telling joke made its first appearance on the hospital wards. The following "gallows humor" remark, made by a chief resident, was recorded during anthropological fieldwork: "Who are the five H's at risk of AIDS?" The answer, told with a half-laugh, goes, "Homosexuals, heroin users, hemophiliacs, Haitians, and *house staff*." House staff, of course, is a shorthand term for medical interns and residents.

At this time concern about the disease was rising among physicians in San Francisco, a city with large numbers of patients, but the disease was as yet "undiscovered" by the general public and the media. Specialty physicians, those oncologists and others who encountered patients very early in the epidemic, experienced a rise in concern earlier than the house officers in the study, that is, at about the beginning of 1982.[7] One survey suggests that even after the period of heightened media attention physicians in general practice were not much concerned about health risks due to AIDS.[8] In the period of time covered by our study, fear seemed to be related to direct exposure to the earliest patients with the disease.

An additional factor in the fear level that summer and early fall was the first report by the Centers for Disease Control of AIDS in four health care workers without other risk factors, published in July.[9] Although confusing, this report was widely discussed. Concern from scientific sources was matched by widely publicized examples of fear. In a much discussed event in June, two Bay Area nurses resigned rather than care for an AIDS patient.[10]

In San Franciso hospitals fear of AIDS was expressed in many ways. There were numerous rumors, including reports that patients with AIDS were refused admission to intensive care units because of physician fear of contagion. Some physicians reportedly refused to perform certain procedures, such as bronchoscopy, in which intimate patient contact is involved. Fear was also expressed indirectly as physicians appeared to shun the newly developed hepatitis B vaccine out of concern that it was obtained from gay male donors at high risk for AIDS.[11] In a climate of fear rumors flourished and anecdotes abounded. Residents were not immune to the public outcry. One stated, "Everyone reads the paper and everyone is a little bit fearful about whether any of us are going to get AIDS."

And finally, throughout this period the geometric expansion in the number of AIDS patients seen in the three UCSF teaching hospitals continued unabated. By the summer of 1983 it was not unusual for AIDS patients to make up 20 percent of the hospitalized patients on the medical service at San Francisco General Hospital. In response to this dramatic increase in patients a specialized AIDS ward was opened in the hospital in July 1983.

## RESIDENT RESPONSE TO AIDS

Faced with an ever increasing number of AIDS patients the residents, along with many early AIDS "watchers," responded with grave concern about the nature and extent of the epidemic. This concern was expressed clearly in the resident interviews. One physician commented, "I'm just sort of dumbfounded at the numbers." Another resident described the AIDS epidemic as the "greatest tragedy of the twentieth century. . . . It's gonna be bad; it's gonna be real bad."

For the physicians caring for AIDS patients on a daily basis the general horror of the epidemic was magnified by the horror of the disease's effects on individual patients. In the interviews, many residents expressed alarm at the devastating nature of the clinical manifestations of AIDS. They used adjectives to describe the illness such as "horrible," "terrible," and "overwhelming." It was described as a "wasting" illness that "overruns the patient." Another stated, "They can't eat, they have continuous diarrhea, and they have . . . fevers constantly; they wither away before your eyes." Dealing with the disease was "frustrating" and "saddening" for the residents.

For the intern, who along with nursing staff comprised the front line of medical care for many hospitalized San Francisco AIDS patients, the clinical reality of AIDS translated into a greatly increased workload. The devastating infections commonplace in AIDS patients require constant vigilance on the part of caregivers. For the intern this means added work. One resident summarized the problem by saying that AIDS patients might comprise 30 percent of the actual patient load but accounted for 90 percent of the resident's work.

Despite fear, anxiety, and an increased workload, many of the residents interviewed responded positively to caring for AIDS patients. Many stated that they enjoyed the "challenge" of a new and difficult disease entity, emphasizing that one couldn't just look up the answers in a textbook. Everything was new and exciting. The positive and intriguing element of the earliest phases of the epidemic was the intellectual challenge presented by the disease AIDS. As the first patients began to appear they had the quality of a mystery or puzzle, eliciting intense excitement and curiosity. While observing on hospital wards, we heard AIDS described as the "greatest thing to hit hem/onc [hematology/oncology] in twenty years." The promise of unlocking the basic relationship between a viral insult, the body's immune response, and the development of cancer was enormously seductive. During ward observations in 1982, when AIDS patients were not yet an everyday part of hospital life, they were treated as the classic "interesting patient." Residents came to daily conferences armed with the latest articles, excited at the prospect of demonstrating their knowledge. Physicians concentrated on diagnosing and treating the myriad unusual infections characteristic of AIDS patients. Successfully treating these infections, many of them previously rare or unfamiliar, was "gratifying."

As the epidemic grew and more and more of the patients the residents were caring for died difficult and horrible deaths, this initial enthusiasm withered. The residents' ideas of what constituted terminal illness were altered by their experience with AIDS. Because of the young age of most patients, physicians found it difficult to consider them "dying patients." One resident said, "We don't want to consider them terminal." Yet, another remarked in frustration, "making the diagnosis is making a terminal diagnosis. . . . They're dying patients with medicine as it is now." The poor prognosis of most patients made decision-making about aggressive versus supportive therapy particularly difficult, especially in the first years of the crisis, when considerable uncertainty about response to particular treatments was the norm. Many residents expressed concern about aggressiveness. One stated that he felt an obligation to do "everything" and yet was sure that if faced with the same options he would "just lie on the beach." The ethical dilemmas of AIDS care continue.[12]

This dimension of AIDS, the constant specter of death, was made more difficult for the residents by the many parallels between the AIDS patients and the residents themselves in social status, education, and age. One informant described the typical AIDS patient as "different than most other patients in the hospital; they're more like *me*." Another resident summed up the many parallels by stating, "They're all your peers." Residents valued the characteristics of AIDS patients that they valued in themselves, particularly intelligence and being well-informed about their disease. Of course, not all residents appreciated these characteristics of AIDS patients. A minority of house officers described the typical AIDS patient as "demanding, aggressive, angry, and bitter."

Unlike some cities where large numbers of patients were intravenous (IV) drug users, the response of residents in our study was influenced by the fact that almost 100 percent of early AIDS cases in San Francisco occurred in gay men. Responses to the questionnaire revealed that the vast majority of the house officers did not regard themselves as gay. Although homophobic responses are difficult to prove either negatively or positively, the responses of residents contained deep concern about this issue. Many lamented the fact that AIDS patients were being "stigmatized." Other physicians mentioned their struggles to accept lifestyles that were "foreign" to them. One resident wrote this eloquent comment on the margin of the questionnaire: "Another positive aspect of working with AIDS patients is learning about the simple humanity of gay men. Stereotypes about fast-lane types and limp-wrists are broken down pretty quickly. Ultimately, I think the AIDS crisis will reduce homophobia amongst physicians."

## SATISFACTION IN CARING FOR AIDS PATIENTS

In the questionnaire, we asked residents about their level of satisfaction in taking care of AIDS patients. One resident responded by circling both extremes, "Dislike Intensely" and "Enjoy Very Much." This response indicates a basic contradiction presented by AIDS. Its care presents a combination of challenge and frustration.

Keeping in mind that all residents probably had mixed reactions to AIDS similar to the one just explained, it is useful to look at the actual questionnaire results. One factor associated with a positive reaction to caring for AIDS patients was the resident's actual experience. Among those who had cared for more than ten patients, 65 percent said they enjoyed caring for AIDS patients. In contrast, only 32 percent of residents who had cared for fewer than ten patients said they enjoyed the work ($p=0.02$).[13] Likewise, the residents' level of training was an important predictor of response to AIDS patients. The percentage of residents stating that they enjoyed caring for AIDS patients was 25, 50, and 67 percent for, respectively, first-, second-, and third-year residents ($p=0.04$). There is almost a complete reversal between first- and third-year residents. Similarly, when asked to rank the desirability of caring for different types of patients (including a cancer patient, someone with chronic lung disease, etc.) residents who had seen the fewest AIDS patients ranked them as least desirable.

## CONCERN ABOUT CONTRACTING AIDS

So far we have not addressed the question of fear; yet it is central to understanding residents' reactions to AIDS. Even though the data were collected after the period of peak fear among residents, our study revealed that significant concern about their own health remained a very real issue for many residents. When asked during the interview to comment on their response to the AIDS epidemic, fully half of the residents *began* their discussion by bringing up the issue of risk to their own health. The issue of risk dominated the discussion despite the general nature of the initial interview question. When asked directly if they had concerns about their own health two-thirds responded affirmatively. Many brought up specific concerns, such as fear of sticking themselves with a contaminated needle and similar accidents. A few residents expressed the belief that it was only a matter of time before a house officer somewhere in the country contracted AIDS.

The questionnaire data confirm the existence of considerable concern among the residents about their own health. Two-thirds of the respondents agreed with the statement that "health workers without other risk factors are at risk of acquiring AIDS." When asked if they had *ever* worried about getting AIDS themselves, the numbers are more striking: 97 percent said that they had worried about contracting AIDS at some point during their residency.

We attempted to evaluate the level of anxiety among residents by asking questions about dreams or suspicious symptoms. A distinct minority of residents, 20 percent, reported that they had experienced symptoms they thought were indicative of AIDS. Twenty percent also reported having dreams or nightmares about AIDS, and 35 percent of the group had worried about giving AIDS to a friend or family member. Finally, 59 percent had worried about the consequences of AIDS for a pregnant resident or other health worker. These findings are consistent with both the interviews and our observations over the year. Dr. Cooke (an attending physician working with the residents in the study) was consulted by a half-dozen residents during the year who were worried about having AIDS.

One interesting finding of the questionnaire study is that men and women appear to differ significantly in their rating of AIDS risk. Among male residents, 84 percent agreed with the statement "health workers without other risk factors are at risk of acquiring AIDS," while only 48 percent of women residents responded affirmatively. The difference in their assessment of risk is striking ($p=0.04$). Not surprisingly, considering their assessment of greater risk, male residents also reported taking greater precautions when caring for AIDS patients. Men reported wearing masks on entering a patient's room (as well as taking other precautions) more frequently than did women (58 percent versus 29 percent; $p=0.03$).

## USE OF PRECAUTIONS

Theoretical concerns about the risk of contracting AIDS become concrete issues when, as a resident, one confronts a patient and must decide about precautions. One resident said:

I *thought* about it a *lot* and I worried about it, but it wasn't: Should I see them or not? It was: How should I protect myself, and how will that interfere with taking care of them? I felt very badly about wearing gloves and gowns and masks because I felt it alienated them. . . . I felt that it interfered with my ability to take care of the patient[s] and relate to them, and it scared them, alienated them, made them feel ostracized, made them feel sicker than they were. So I worried about that.

The use of precautions was complicated by lack of firm knowledge about the exact mode of transmission of the disease. In the early part of the epidemic "official" recommendations changed frequently. Uncertainty complicated the picture. One resident said, "I really don't agree with everyone's saying 'Oh, it's OK' . . . because basically we don't know how it's spread."

Finding some means of protecting oneself is a universal response to fear. We make use of available technology—regardless of firm knowledge of its effectiveness. The leather costume of the European plague doctor may have actually afforded some protection. Although we are more used to the current era's protective garb—gowns, masks, caps, rubber gloves, and occasionally goggles—to the patient there is probably little difference. The costume carries a potent symbolic message: fear of contagion. Many residents were disturbed by this increased distance; some lamented the loss involved in not touching the patient.

When asked in the questionnaire about their "typical" use of precautions, most residents reported quite rational use of protective gear: 92 percent reported wearing gloves while drawing blood, recommended then as now; 83 percent did not wear a gown during routine contact. In other types of precaution, such as use of masks, a practice not usually recommended, there was more variability in response, an outlet for the expression of fear.

## THE NATURE OF RESPONSIBILITY

Despite the fairly high levels of concern about AIDS among the medical residents, there was also a very clear expression of a sense of obligation to care for AIDS patients regardless of personal fear or any particular patient characteristics. To our knowledge, with the exception of pregnant residents, no house officer ever refused to care for an AIDS patient. When asked on the questionnaire if they had heard of fellow residents attempting to avoid the care of AIDS patients, two-thirds of the sample responded that they had heard of *no* house officers refusing to care for an AIDS patient. The one-third of residents who had heard of colleagues attempting to avoid or refuse AIDS patients indicated that they knew of only one or two examples. When asked if medical personnel should have the theoretical option of refusing to care for AIDS patients, two-thirds of the residents answered negatively, expressing the idea that refusal should not be a choice. The earliest published recommendations came to the same basic conclusion.[14]

Likewise, the interview data reveal a very clear sense of responsibility to the patient with AIDS. When questioned directly about how they viewed their responsibility, the overwhelming response from residents was that their responsibilities to AIDS patients were identical to those of any other seriously ill patient. A minority of residents expressed the idea of *greater* responsibility to patients with AIDS because of their young age and the devastating nature of the illness with its extensive social, as well as purely medical, needs. One resident invoked the Hippocratic Oath, stating, "I think part of that is to treat every patient, no matter if you are a little afraid that you might catch something." This notion of a basic obligation to treat all patients was a dominant theme. When asked directly if they would consider refusing to care for an AIDS patient the characteristic response was, "No. I just worry about it. I would never do that. It just wouldn't seem right to me."

Some residents brought up the difficult question of whether they would perform mouth-to-mouth resuscitation on an AIDS patient, perhaps the most extreme case of conflict between self versus other. A few stated that they would be "incredibly loath to mouth-to-mouth." This issue raised feelings of both guilt and anger. One resident, after stating fear and unwillingness to make the "ultimate sacrifice," immediately expressed guilt about this admission. Another expressed anger that residents were expected to take all risks without complaint, stating, "It's the whole macho physician thing. . . . *You* [the physician] don't matter. . . . You're expendable."

## STRUCTURAL ISSUES IN RESIDENT TRAINING

Lest the reader think we are attempting to paint an overly heroic picture of the UCSF residents, it is necessary to point out that outright refusal to accept a patient assignment would be an extremely difficult, and visible, act for a medical resident. The structural constraints of the house staff training program are a serious consideration. The level of conformity and discipline (as well as commitment) is almost militaristic. Other, particularly senior, physicians, are not merely colleagues; they are also constantly evaluating the residents' performance. These evaluations, and one's eventual "reputation" as a resident, are crucial in either opening or closing later career possibilities. As Charles Bosk[15] has pointed out, a resident's *moral* failings are much more serious than any technical error in procedure or medical knowledge. The latter are all potentially correctible; the former are serious and unforgivable. Hence, according to Bosk, moral errors are given much more weight in evaluating physicians in training. Therefore, actual refusal to care for an AIDS patient may not have been a realistic option for the residents.

It is also important to point out that AIDS patients are an addition to an already stressful and demanding training period. They must be fitted into workweeks that frequently average well over 100 hours. If residents seem heroic in their expressions of responsibility (or were simply not able to refuse AIDS care), they were certainly not hesitant to complain. I have already mentioned that a big concern was the additional burden of work caused by the demanding clinical care of AIDS patients. One resident complained, "I feel so whipped by them." This additional burden created the danger of an "us against them" atmosphere.

One complaint that surfaced fairly early in the epidemic (and was more recently expressed as a "Sounding Board" in the *New England Journal of Medicine* by a UCSF resident)[16] is the effect of AIDS on the quality of the residents' education. In the interviews some residents complained that their education was being harmed by the necessity of "being an AIDS doctor." One resident joked that his knowledge of dermatology was limited to "poison oak and Kaposi's sarcoma." There were also complaints about the "once a month grand rounds on AIDS." One said, "I worry about my education. . . . I wish I knew more about pneumococcal pneumonia and less about AIDS."

Another source of complaints for some residents was the lack of appreciation for what they saw as their enormous efforts with AIDS patients. In San Francisco the media have paid considerable attention to AIDS, including extensive coverage of the health professionals involved in caring for patients. From the residents' point of view, the one group missing from this extensive media attention has been interns and residents—health professionals who do much of the hands-on work with patients, especially once they are hospitalized. One resident mentioned that they were the one group noticeably absent from the reports about the opening of the AIDS ward at San Francisco General Hospital. The resident complained that the house staff did the work and the others got the glory—the nurses from the AIDS ward received press attention and were celebrated as heroes and the more senior attending physicians were building highly visible and successful scientific careers on the basis of their AIDS research. The image of the lowly, unsung resident or intern who does the "scut work" but does not share in any of the glory is perhaps a bit overstated here but does contain an element of truth.

During the period of our study this problem was accentuated (for some residents) by a perception of abandonment and unshared risk. Some residents complained that they were given very little assistance with the medical management of extremely ill AIDS patients. One said:

I felt that there were too many people standing around pontificating about it . . . I.D. [infectious disease] people here, pulmonary people there . . . everyone standing around scratching their heads, and then they all go *home* at night— leaving me with this patient with all his family needs, and emotional and psychiatric needs, and their fevers, and their weight loss, and throwing up and their diarrhea. And not knowing what to do and . . . everyone leaving. It was like there was too much intellectualizing and not enough support. . . . It made me really *angry*.

The idea of the resident as unsung hero extended to the area of possible risk of contracting AIDS. During the early part of the epidemic the residents felt compelled to perform the work that other occupational groups refused to do. One resident commented on the "phobia" that existed:

People are so afraid . . . at this point. [AIDS patients] get their meals on paper plates, the dieticians won't walk in with their trays, the blood drawers won't draw their blood and the nurses don't want to take their temperatures. . . . They get treated more as lepers than anything else. It's aggravating, [and] then the intern has to do all this. The intern has to do everything that is normally someone else's job because everyone else is afraid of catching something—which I don't think can happen. But, again, [it's] ironic that even if you could catch something it wouldn't matter because [resident laughs] there is always an intern there to do your job.

## CONCLUSION

What do these data mean? In trying to account for the different responses of male and female residents to AIDS we have no definitive answers but would like to offer some speculations. First, it seems possible that women as a group may be less affected by "homophobic" considerations in caring for AIDS patients. Less personally threatened by homosexuality, women may simply be more comfortable with the patients and consequently less afraid. A second, related possibility is that male residents may have experienced greater fear and anxiety in caring for AIDS patients because of a more intense identification with the patients, many of whom were almost identical to the residents in terms of age, education, and general background. The constant contact with men close to their own age, dying from a horrible disease, might have caused fear and anxiety to intensify. Women may simply be one step removed from this level of fear.

We do not wish to create the impression that these differences in response are the crucial issue. In reality, all residents are affected by the same underlying dynamic—balancing concern for self with responsibility to patients. This is seen more clearly in the changes in the response to AIDS patients that occur during medical training. Somehow, physicians were able to accommodate themselves to the intense fear many encountered on first caring for AIDS patients. Satisfaction in caring for AIDS patients increased. How can we account for this? Is it explained simply (and cynically) by increasing clinical expertise and reduced physical contact with the patient as one accrues seniority? We think it is part of a more fundamental process that occurs in medical education.

Albert Jonsen has suggested in an essay called "Watching the Doctor" that a profound moral paradox pervades the practice of medicine.[17] He suggests that this paradox arises from conflict between the two most basic principles of morality: self-interest and altruism. We were both perplexed and intrigued when first analyzing our study results to see this paradox running through almost every resident's comments like a rich vein of silver—to be unearthed and then reflected upon. The residents' struggles are clear. They are abstract and general (how do you balance fear of acquiring AIDS against a feeling of duty to care for all patients?) and quite specific (do you wear a mask when risk is uncertain or do you enter the patient's room without protection, consciously attempting to avoid stigmatizing him?). The struggles are also personal (do you focus on the intellectual thrills of AIDS or attempt to meet the patient's enormous need for social and emotional attention?). Each physician confronts these questions and gradually forges a personal answer, an answer informed and shaped by the intense stresses of training. Most are able to overcome fear and care for patients. Learning the proper balance is a key moral task of training.

With the AIDS epidemic the conflict between altruism and self-interest has regained a measure of clarity that seemed lost in the scientific achievements of the postwar antibiotic era. The residents in our study—indeed, most of their physician teachers—had not confronted the polio epidemics of the 1950s, the most recent reminder of our vulnerability.

With the advent of AIDS we have been vividly reminded of a fact central to medical practice.

## ACKNOWLEDGMENTS

The authors wish to thank Margaret Wrensch and Karen Vranison for assistance with the statistical analysis. We are also indebted to the medical residents who—in spite of enormous demands on their time—generously agreed to participate in the study on which this chapter is based.

## NOTES

1. P. Klass. The age-old fear of contagion arises when treating an AIDS patient. *New York Times* (October 25, 1984).

2. The interview study was part of a larger anthropological study of medical house officer's care of dying patients (see note 3). This research was supported by the James Picker Foundation, the Maureen Church Coburn Charitable Trust, and the University of California, San Francisco (Academic Senate Committee on Research and the Research, Evaluation, and Allocation Committee, School of Medicine).

3. J. H. Muller and B. A. Koenig. On the boundary of life and death: The definition of dying by medical residents. In *Biomedicine Examined*, ed. M. Lock and D. Gordon. Boston: D. Reidel. Forthcoming.

4. See H. E. Varmus. This volume, Chapter 1.

5. E. McCray et al. Occupational risk of the acquired immunodeficiency syndrome among health care workers. *New England Journal of Medicine* 314 (1986): 1127–32.

6. Richard Harris of the *San Francisco Examiner* assisted in obtaining this information.

7. This statement is based on our observation of events in San Francisco and may not reflect the situation elsewhere in the United States.

8. E. Barrett-Connor. Physician knowledge and concerns about AIDS. *Western Journal of Medicine* 140 (1984):652–53.

9. Centers for Disease Control. An evaluation of the acquired immunodeficiency syndrome (AIDS) reported in health-care personnel—United States. *Morbidity and Mortality Weekly Reports* 32 (1983):358–60.

10. Two RNs refuse to treat AIDS patient, resign. *San Francisco Examiner* (June 12, 1983).

11. A. M. Schwartz and T. L. Chorba. Hepatitis vaccine and the acquired immunodeficiency syndrome (letter). *Annals of Internal Medicine* 99 (1983):567–68.

12. R. Steinbrook et al. Ethical dilemmas in caring for patients with the acquired immunodeficiency syndrome. *Annals of Internal Medicine* 103 (1985):787–90. A. R. Jonsen, M. Cooke, and B. A. Koenig. AIDS and ethics. *Issues in Science and Technology* 2 (1986):56–65.

13. The $p$ values are included to indicate that the difference between the two responses cited was statistically significant and not simply the result of chance.

Statistical significance was assessed using a chi-square test in this and the following comparisons.

14. S. M. Finegold. Protecting health personnel. In *The AIDS Epidemic*, ed. K. Cahill. New York: St. Martin's Press, 1983, pp. 123–36. J. E. Conte et al. Infection-control guidelines for patients with the acquired immunodeficiency syndrome (AIDS). *New England Journal of Medicine* 309 (1983):740–44.

15. C. L. Bosk. *Forgive and Remember: Managing Medical Failure*. Chicago: University of Chicago Press, 1979.

16. R. M. Wachter. The impact of the acquired immunodeficiency syndrome on medical residency training. *New England Journal of Medicine* 314 (1986):177–80.

17. A. R. Jonsen. Watching the doctor. *New England Journal of Medicine* 308 (1983):1531–35.

# 9 LIFE-SUSTAINING TREATMENT IN PATIENTS WITH AIDS: CHALLENGES TO TRADITIONAL DECISION MAKING
*Bernard Lo*

Because AIDS is presently a fatal disease, decisions about life-sustaining treatment frequently must be made. These decisions are especially difficult because patients with AIDS are painfully like their caregivers. Often they are young, well educated, and previously healthy. One medical resident said, "Telling a patient he has AIDS is like giving your brother a death sentence." Dilemmas about life-sustaining treatment for patients with AIDS will become even more frequent as the epidemic continues. In the next five years, 10 to 20 percent of the 1 million to 2 million people who are already infected with HIV virus are expected to develop clinical manifestations of AIDS.[1] In other words, 100,000 to 400,000 more persons will develop AIDS even if no further individuals are infected.

An ethical, legal, and medical consensus recommends that decisions about medical care, including decisions about life-sustaining treatment, be made jointly by physicians and informed, competent patients or the surrogates of incompetent patients.[2] This principle is supported by court rulings, by the recommendations of a presidential commission, and by articles in the medical literature. Competent patients should give informed consent or refusal to treatments recommended by physicians. They can refuse treatments even if such refusal shortens their life or if their physicians, families, and friends regard their refusal as unwise or foolish. Patient preferences may be especially important in a new disease like AIDS. Some patients may want maximal care, hoping for a therapeutic breakthrough, while others do not consider a small possibility of benefit to be worth the potential pain and difficulty of intensive care.

But patients or their representatives cannot demand whatever care they wish from physicians. For instance, physicians should not accede to patient requests for direct killing, such as committing active euthanasia or abetting a suicide.[3] Moreover, as I shall discuss later, physicians are not obligated to give care that is futile or that will not benefit the patient.

Analyzing dilemmas about life-sustaining treatment will not only improve the care of patients with AIDS but also illuminate four important problems with the conventional approach to these ethical problems: First, patient preferences about life-sustaining treatment may not be informed. Second, it may be difficult for caregivers to decide whether treatment is futile. Third, the apparent scarcity of health care resources may limit treatment. Fourth, families of incompetent patients may not be appropriate surrogate decision makers.

## INFORMED DECISIONS BY COMPETENT PATIENTS

To be able to give informed consent or refusal, the patient must understand the medical situation. Specifically, the patient should appreciate the risks and benefits of the proposed treatment, the alternatives, and the consequences of his decision. Our research at UCSF, however, shows that patients with AIDS overestimate the effectiveness of life-sustaining treatment.

Researchers interviewed 118 homosexual men with AIDS who were receiving outpatient care at San Francisco General Hospital and at the University of California at San Francisco about their preferences for life-sustaining treatment.[4] Nationally, about three-quarters of AIDS cases occur in homosexual or bisexual men; in San Francisco, the proportion is over 90 percent. We were particularly interested in their preferences about treatment for pneumocystis pneumonia, the most common opportunistic infection in AIDS and a frequent cause of death. In severe cases, decisions must be made regarding intensive care with intubation and mechanical ventilation. About three-quarters of the patients in our study had thought about such life-sustaining treatment, wanted to discuss these issues with their physicians, and had preferences about *what* treatment they would want and *whom* they wanted to make decisions if they were unable to do so. In other words, these patients wanted to play an active role in decisions.

But the patients overestimated the usefulness of mechanical ventilation in severe pneumocystic pneumonia. We asked them to estimate the prognosis of patients with AIDS and pneumocystis who required mechanical ventilation. The numerical mean of their estimates of the survival rate with that procedure was 53 percent. There was a wide range of estimates: About a third of the respondents estimated that over 75 percent of such patients survived; almost one-half estimated that between 50 percent and 75 percent of patients left the hospital alive. But research has shown that the *actual* survival of such patients after mechanical ventilation is 14 percent.[5] This rate has been reported by several AIDS referral centers and has not improved over the past few years. Our findings are particularly surprising since our subjects were well educated and lived in San Francisco, where AIDS is widely discussed in the media. Even patients who might be expected to be knowledgeable were not. Patients who actually had pneumocystis, who had been hospitalized during the past year, or who knew someone who died from AIDS were no more realistic than others.

These findings raise serious concerns about shared decision making. Consent or refusal based on inaccurate medical facts is not informed. Good ethical decisions must be based on accurate medical information. We do not know whether patients would change their preferences about life-sustaining treatment if their estimates of its effectiveness were more realistic.

We do *not* believe that our study implies that we should abandon the ideal of informed consent as impractical. But our findings dramatize the need to improve communication between caregivers and patients and to improve patient education. As caregivers, we cannot assume that our patients understand the basic medical information. Nor can we rely on the media, other caregivers, or volunteer counselors to inform patients. We must anticipate common misconceptions and discuss them explicitly with individual patients.

## MEDICALLY FUTILE TREATMENT

Shared decision making is problematic not only because patient preferences may not be informed, but also because of difficulties with determining whether treatment is futile. Physicians have no ethical, medical, or legal obligation to provide treatment that will not benefit the patient, even if the patient or the patient's surrogate requests it.[6] The abstract principle that futile treatment need not be given evokes little disagreement. But problems may occur in deciding what particular treatments are "futile."

In the strictest sense, treatment is futile if the patient is moribund and will die within hours or days regardless of what treatment is given. An example is a patient with AIDS and pneumocystis pneumonia who is receiving intensive care with antibiotics and mechanical ventilation but who is becoming increasingly hypoxic. Further treatment in this situation would be futile, since the likelihood of survival is nil. In addition, it would be misleading and unrealistic to offer cardiopulmonary resuscitation as a therapeutic option. But in other situations, caregivers may use the term "futility" in a looser sense.

Controversy over whether treatment is futile may occur for several reasons.[7] First, medical knowledge may be incorrect. Physicians sometimes declare that it is inappropriate to place an AIDS patient with pneumocystis on a ventilator because to do so is futile. The medical literature, however, does not support such a gloomy prognosis. As already mentioned, 14 percent of patients with pneumocystis pneumonia who are placed on mechanical ventilation are discharged alive from the hospital.

Second, judgments about an individual case may be incorrect. We do not know how long a trial of antibiotics is necessary before further treatment can be considered futile. On the one hand, most physicians would agree that if a patient had not responded to antibiotics after one or two days, it would be premature to consider further treatment futile. On the other hand, if pneumocystis had progressed despite three weeks of therapy with both of the antibiotics usually effective against this infection, most clinicians would consider further treatment futile. Between these two extremes, we must depend on clinical judgment, which is fallible. Good ethical decisions require caregivers as well as patients to have correct medical facts in order to be able to make sound, well-informed clinical judgments. In a new disease like AIDS, accurate medical information may be changing rapidly or be difficult to obtain.

Third, claims that treatment is futile entail value judgments as well as scientific knowledge. As physicians we may be tempted to reduce ethical dilemmas to technical questions that can be decided objectively. It clearly requires scientific expertise to know that the survival of patients with AIDS and pneumocystis who require mechanical ventilation is 14 percent. But interpreting whether a treatment with a 14 percent probability of success, or a 1.4 percent or a 0.14 percent probability of success, is futile requires a value judgment. Under the principle of shared decision making, that value judgment should be made by patients, not by the caregivers.

Fourth, judgments about futility may actually be policy decisions about allocating health care resources. Projections about the AIDS epidemic raise fears that the cost of caring for patients with AIDS will overwhelm the health care system. Nationally it costs an average of $147,000 to care for each patient with AIDS.[8] If 400,000 more patients develop AIDS in the next five years, the cost will be almost $60 billion. Some suggest that the country must restrict the treatment of patients with AIDS, so that resources will be available to treat patients with other diseases. In particular, some question whether spending money for expensive life-sustaining treatment for AIDS patients is appropriate.

## ALLOCATING HEALTH CARE RESOURCES

On one level, allocation decisions may be made at the bedside by physicians. At busy hospitals, physicians often consider the availability of scarce resources like intensive care beds or caregiver time. Doctors can respond to modest resource constraints on a case-by-case basis without adversely affecting patient outcomes.[9] They may adjust the threshold for admitting patients to the intensive care unit or for transferring them out of the intensive care unit. Or they may use the emergency room or postoperative recovery room temporarily as an intensive care unit. Such decisions use medical resources more efficiently without withholding care that might benefit patients. The likelihood of harming a patient by withholding treatments of marginal or no benefit is small. Thus it seems reasonable to leave such decisions to physicians.

But other decisions to allocate scarce resources would withhold treatments that might benefit patients. An example would be policy to withhold mechanical ventilation from all patients with AIDS and pneumocystis. Such decisions require social choices that should be made through the political process, not at the bedside.

At the bedside, it may appear that the only solution to the problem of scarce resources is to limit treatments. But from a political or social perspective, other alternatives may be possible.[10] If there is a shortage of intensive care beds, regional planning may be helpful. The majority of cases of AIDS occur in metropolitan regions with a surplus of acute hospital and intensive care beds. If one hospital has too many patients with AIDS who require intensive care beds, arrangements might be made to admit patients to other hospitals. If the problem is insufficient funding for a public hospital, political lobbying might increase appropriations for the care of patients with AIDS.

Furthermore, costs might be reduced in ways that are more ethically, politically, and medically acceptable than rationing expensive but useful life-sustaining treatment. In San Francisco, the cost of caring for a patient with AIDS is under $28,000, less than one-fifth the national average cost.[11] These savings are possible because of the availability of outpatient and hospice care, educational programs, volunteer counseling, and legal and housing assistance.

It is difficult to justify restricting the care of patients with AIDS for economic reasons unless society is also willing to restrict the care of other patients with similar prognoses. Our sense of justice would be violated if we did not treat similar groups of patients in the same manner.[12] If the public is unwilling to debate allocation decisions openly, some groups of patients may face discrimination. Homosexual men with AIDS, who already are subjected to discrimination in employment and housing, fear further injustice.

## DECISION MAKING FOR INCOMPETENT PATIENTS

The care of AIDS patients also illustrates problems with decisions regarding incompetent patients. Patients with AIDS may be incompetent when decisions about life-sustaining treatment must be made for a variety of reasons, including direct invasion of the brain by the HIV virus, opportunistic infections involving the central nervous system, or metabolic problems caused by severe lack of oxygen.

How should decisions be made for incompetent patients? Two questions must be answered: What criteria should be used and who should make decisions. There is an ethical, legal, and medical consensus that the previously stated wishes of the patient should guide decisions for incompetent patients. If these wishes are unclear or unknown, the best interests of the patient should be followed.[13]

Traditionally, physicians ask families of incompetent patients to act as surrogates. But this tradition may not be appropriate for homosexual men with AIDS. Many gay men want their partners or lovers to make decisions for them, not members of their biological family. They believe that their partners know their preferences or interests better than their families do. The conflict between patients and families was illustrated poignantly by a case in our study.[14] The parents of one patient wrote that AIDS was God's punishment for his homosexuality.

In some states, competent patients can take steps to ensure that their preferences about care will be respected if they become incompetent. In California, the durable power of attorney for health care is the most flexible and comprehensive way for competent patients to make advance plans for their care.[15] A gay patient with AIDS may designate his partner to act as a surrogate decision maker if he should become incompetent. But in most states, the law is unclear or silent about decisions for incompetent patients. Most states do not have specific statutes authorizing the durable power of attorney for health care or the designation of a proxy decision maker. In these states, the partner, friend, or lover of an incompetent patient may have no legal standing to make surrogate decisions. The patient cannot be sure that his preferences will be followed, and caregivers cannot be assured of legal immunity if they follow the patient's previously expressed wishes. Caregivers may feel trapped if the family and partner of a homosexual man disagree. Respecting the patient's previously stated preferences, which is appropriate from an ethical and medical perspective, may subject the caregiver to legal risk.

In summary, the AIDS epidemic creates difficult dilemmas about life-sustaining treatment. As caregivers we must try to resolve these dilemmas in a humane and fair way. One patient in our study expressed eloquently the importance of maintaining his dignity in this tragic situation: "I hope physicians everywhere will remember that they are dealing with real people and not with plastic dolls they can manipulate at whim. I am frightened, but not of death. Rather, I am frightened of being helpless."[16] Although physicians are not yet able to alter the course of this fatal disease, they can offer their patients comfort and respect their patients' humanity.

## ACKNOWLEDGMENTS

This work was supported in part by grants from the University of California Task Force on AIDS and from the James Picker Foundation. I wish to thank Robert Steinbrook, Paul Volberding, Harry Hollander, and Jeff Moulton for their collaboration and assistance.

## NOTES

1. S. Staver. Nation's AIDS epidemic triggers insurance woes for millions of people. *American Medical News* (April 11, 1986):1.

2. *In the matter of Claire C. Conroy*, 486 A 2d 1209 (N.J. 1985). *Barber v. Superior Court of State of California*, 195 Cal Rptr. 484, 147 Cal. App. 3d 1054 (1983). President's Commission for the Study of Ethical Problems in Medicine and Biomedical and Behavioral Research. *Deciding to Forego Life-Sustaining Treatment.* Washington, D.C.: U.S. Government Printing Office, 1983. B. Lo and A. R. Jonsen. Clinical decisions to limit treatment. *Annals of Internal Medicine* 93 (1980): 764–68. A. R. Jonsen, M. Siegler, and W. J. Winslade. *Clinical Ethics.* New York: Macmillan, 1982, pp. 109–24.

3. R. M. Veatch. *A Theory of Medical Ethics.* New York: Basic Books, 1981, pp. 177–89.

4. R. Steinbrook et al. Preferences of homosexual men with the acquired immunodeficiency syndrome for life-sustaining treatment. *New England Journal of Medicine* 314 (1986):457–60.

5. J. F. Murray et al. Pulmonary complications of the acquired immunodeficiency syndrome. *New England Journal of Medicine* 310 (1984):1682–88. R. M. Wachter et al. Intensive care of patients with the acquired immunodeficiency syndrome. *American Review of Respiratory Disease* 134 (1986):891–96.

6. R. Steinbrook et al. Ethical dilemmas in caring for patients with the acquired immunodeficiency syndrome. *Annals of Internal Medicine* 103 (1985):787–90 and Lo and Jonsen, Clinical decisions.

7. Steinbrook et al., Ethical dilemmas.

8. A. M. Hardy et al. The economic impact of the first 10,000 cases of acquired immunodeficiency syndrome in the United States. *Journal of the American Medical Association* 255 (1986):209–11.

9. M. J. Strauss et al. Rationing of intensive care unit services: An everyday occurrence. *Journal of the American Medical Association* 255 (1986):1143–46 and see Steinbrook et al., Ethical dilemmas.

10. See Steinbrook et al., Ethical dilemmas.

11. A. A. Scitovsky and D. P. Rice. Estimates of the direct and indirect costs of

acquired immunodeficiency syndrome in the United States, 1985, 1986, and 1991. *Public Health Reports* 102 (1987):5-7.

12. Jonsen, Siegler, and Winslade, *Clinical Ethics* and Veatch, *Theory of Medical Ethics*.

13. *In the matter of Claire C. Conroy*; President's Commission, *Life-Sustaining Treatment*; Lo and Jonsen, Clinical decisions; and Jonsen, Siegler, and Winslade, *Clinical Ethics*.

14. Steinbrook et al., Preferences of homosexual men.

15. R. Steinbrook and B. Lo. Decision making for incompetent patients by designated proxy. *New England Journal of Medicine* 310 (1984):1598-601.

16. Steinbrook et al., Preferences of homosexual men.

# 10 LAW, ETHICS, AND ADVANCE DIRECTIVES REGARDING THE MEDICAL CARE OF AIDS PATIENTS

*Lawrence J. Nelson*

As AIDS currently is a progressive, incurable, and invariably fatal disease, both AIDS patients and their physicians and other professionals involved in their medical care must make decisions about the ethically acceptable and legally proper course of treatment these patients will undergo. While individual episodes of opportunistic infection or malignancy often can be successfully treated, the underlying disease of the immune system cannot. Here or there a therapeutic battle can be won, but the war for preserving the patient's life will tragically, and invariably, be lost. Consequently, decisions will inevitably have to be made about whether or not to employ an experimental therapy, whether or not to use mechanical ventilation, whether or not to resuscitate in the event of cardiac or respiratory arrest.

## SOLICITING PATIENTS' PREFERENCES

Given that these decisions must be made, how are they to be made? The readily apparent and most commonly suggested answer is that decisions are to be made by the patient in conjunction with the physician. Given the progressive and incurable nature of AIDS and the fact that many AIDS patients will at some point need treatments such as mechanical ventilation or cardiopulmonary resuscitation, professionals who care for AIDS patients, particularly physicians, should actively solicit the patient's own wishes regarding the future course of treatment in a sensitive but direct way and discuss the future use of life-sustaining treatment.[1] Clinicians not infrequently find this to be an unpleasant task that they would rather avoid. It is not surprising that those dedicated to caring for and curing the ill experience profound difficulty when talking to their patients about their inability to save them from what, in the case of AIDS, is usually the untimely death of a young person. Nonetheless, it is the clinician's responsibility to make plans with the AIDS patients about their future treatment.

As in all such clinical situations, the solicitation of AIDS patients' views about their future course of treatment should be done at a time and by a person or persons appropriate to the patients' circumstances. In some cases, it may be best to postpone engaging the patient in a direct discussion of future treatment plans until such time as it is clear that the patient's prognosis is worsening and that definite choices will soon have to be made about how aggressive and invasive further treatment will be. Similarly, some patients may be better served by discussing these plans with a nurse, a social worker, a member of the clergy, or a counselor—either in direct conjunction with or in lieu of the patient's attending physician. However, the use of discretion in approaching AIDS patients about their preferences regarding life-sustaining treatment should not collapse into procrastination. The tragedy of AIDS is only heightened if clinicians fail to elicit and follow as best they can a patient's own views about the course of the remainder of his or her life and of the possible circumstances of the patient's death.

The obligation of the clinician to discuss the use of life-sustaining treatment with patients is obviously rooted in a conviction that the best plan of medical treatment for an adult patient will be consonant with that patient's own particular values and desires and that the best way to determine this plan is to consult the patient directly. Speculating about or making inferences about the patient's values and desires at a later time when the primary source of this critical information may be unavailable is not wise. Similarly, it is unwise to discuss future treatment plans with patients using only euphemisms such as "heroic treatment," "extraordinary measures," "artificial means," or even "life-sustaining treatment," since these phrases may mean very different things to clinician and patient.

Decisions regarding the fate of seriously ill AIDS patients are simply too important to be based upon misunderstanding, false assumptions, or mistaken perceptions. Consequently, it is prudent for clinicians to discuss in a forthright manner the future use of specific treatments that may be needed to preserve the patient's life. Mechanical ventilation, for example, is one specific treatment that many AIDS patients may need. One recent study reported that the survival rate of AIDS patients with pneumocystis pneumonia who require intubation is only 14 percent.[2] Given that they face those odds and the possibly unpleasant specter of dying in the hospital while intubated, AIDS patients deserve an opportunity to participate in decisions regarding the use of mechanical ventilation after being accurately informed of the situation which they may soon face.

If an adult AIDS patient is legally and ethically competent (that is, able to demonstrate an understanding of the nature of the situation and of the consequences of the choices to be made) and clearly refuses treatment at the time the treatment is offered or in advance, physicians and others should honor that decision. Both common and constitutional law protects the patient's choice even if he or she is not fully lucid or oriented and even if the reasons for refusal make little or no sense to the clinician.[3] Ethically, others are bound to respect the exercise of another person's only human and imperfect freedom even if they do not agree with the exercise of that freedom or do not understand the motives that animate it. Nonetheless, this is not to say that clinicians do not have the responsibility to discuss the matter with such a patient, to attempt to dissuade the patient from what may be a questionable choice, or perhaps even to resign from the patient's care if they cannot in good conscience participate in the patient's decision.[4]

## THE ROLE OF THE FAMILY

However, many AIDS patients become mentally incompetent during the course of their illness and are unable to communicate at the time when important clinical decisions must be made.[5] Traditionally, medicine has turned to the patient's family for guidance and consent about treatment in these situations for two basic reasons. First, family members are presumed to be in the best position to know the patient's values and desires and to be those personally closest to the patient. Second (but given the medical profession's perception of the present malpractice climate, perhaps it should be first), clinicians think they are less likely to run afoul of the long arm of the law if they follow the family's wishes about continuing or discontinuing treatment. Many AIDS patients, however, want a lover or a friend, not family members, to make treatment decisions on their behalf with their physicians when they become incompetent. The central problem with the implementation of such a preference is that the lover or friend has no recognized legal standing to make such decisions. As a practical matter, most physicians and hospitals are going to be very reluctant to follow the directions of a patient's lover or a friend, given the latter's lack of legal authority, particularly if the patient's family is present and opposes the wishes of the lover or friend.

Curiously and ironically, in most states, family members have *no* express legal standing to make such decisions either, but they have at least some de facto authority, if only because family members will usually have standing to sue for the patient's wrongful death.[6] A serious problem with the practice of having a patient's family make treatment decisions for incompetent relatives can be readily seen when members of the family disagree with one another. Except in those very few states with statutes that establish a hierarchy of authority among family members, there is simply no definitive way to determine who speaks for the patient when family members disagree. Many hospital attorneys will advise that in cases in which family members disagree about forgoing treatment of their incompetent relative, the patient must continue receiving treatment until agreement is reached or a court order resolving the disagreement is obtained.

## THE DURABLE POWER OF ATTORNEY
## FOR HEALTH CARE

In one state, however, there is a solution to the problem of determining who has the legal authority to make decisions for an incompetent adult patient. In California, adults can execute a durable power of attorney for health care that confers legal recognition on their appointment of another person to make health care decisions on their behalf when they become incompetent.[7] For all legal purposes regarding most treatment decisions (exceptions include abortion, psychosurgery, and sterilization), the agent has full authority to give or refuse informed consent to treatment on behalf of the patient. The California law permits the patient to state his or her exact wishes about treatment in the document that appoints the agent, and the agent is bound to follow those wishes and any other wishes expressed by the patient in any fashion. As the agent is expressly granted priority over any other person in making health care decisions on behalf of the patient, the patient can specifically designate the one person who is to make treatment decisions, whether that one person be friend, lover, spouse, or family member. The directions of the agent are generally legally binding, even if the agent is not a family member and even if the patient's family disagrees with the agent. Any clinician or provider who in good faith honors a decision of the agent is immunized from any criminal prosecution, civil liability, or professional disciplinary action for so doing.

In short, a durable power of attorney for health care established by statute gives AIDS and other patients an easily utilized and practical means of ensuring that their wishes regarding medical treatment, including the use of life-sustaining procedures, will be made known by a person of their own choosing and, hopefully, honored by their providers as if they themselves had made the decision. Clinicians should be familiar with the durable power of attorney for health care when it is in effect and assist AIDS patients in utilizing it to effectuate their wishes and values regarding treatment of a disease for which there is as yet no cure.

Unfortunately, there are published reports that even in California the durable power of attorney for health care is not widely used by AIDS patients who in fact want their lovers or friends to be substitute decision makers.[8] In the majority of states that do not expressly recognize the durable power of attorney for health care, physicians and other health care professionals should seriously consider actively lobbying for such legislation. Both they and their patients would gain by the enactment of such a law. Patients would remain in control of their bodies and medical fates through their agents. The physician would be able to turn for guidance in making the necessary treatment decisions to a single designated person with clear legal authority to act on the patient's behalf.

In one recent study of 118 homosexual male outpatients with AIDS in San Francisco, 47 percent of the patients wanted their partners or friends to act as substitute decision makers if they became incompetent, 32 percent wanted family members, and 14 percent wanted their physicians.[9] For the reasons mentioned above, the durable power of attorney for health care would be especially important to the 47 percent who wanted their partner or friend to act on their behalf. Interestingly, the California durable-power-of-attorney law would not permit the appointment of the patient's attending physician as agent under any circumstances.[10] If the patients really wanted their physician to make decisions regarding the use of life-sustaining treatment, they would have to appoint a third person as agent and instruct that individual to defer to the physician's recommendations. The 32 percent who wanted family members to act on their behalf in any event would profit from the use of the durable power principally if they wanted to appoint a particular relative as their agent or if they wanted the agent to be guided by certain wishes that could be clearly expressed by the patient in the appointing document itself.

## INSTRUCTIONAL DIRECTIVES

Despite the decided advantages of a statutorily recognized durable power of attorney for health care, it is not the only way for patients to issue advance directives about their care. At least two courts have suggested that clinicians can follow an adult's written advance directive about medical treatment in certain circumstances without fear of adverse legal consequences.[11] Therefore, even in the majority of states that do not expressly recognize the durable power of attorney for health care, persons can still make their wishes known in this manner and should be encouraged to do so by the clinicians caring for them.

There is a significant legal and ethical problem that at least some clinicians have faced with AIDS and other patients who have given advance directives about their care. What does the physician do in the case of patients who requested, or even demanded, at some point in the past that *everything* be done to treat them until death? Does this obligate the physician to initiate cardiopulmonary resuscitation for a now demented AIDS patient who has not much longer to live in any event? In their legitimate desire to give their AIDS patients some hope and comfort, physicians may sometimes promise "to do everything medically" for a patient, but later find themselves questioning the validity of this promise when the treatment they can offer only prolongs a dying process that is not necessarily comfortable or peaceful. On the one hand, it seems legitimate for a patient to ask to be given a chance to live as long as possible. On the other hand, it seems equally legitimate that physicians should not be legally or ethically obligated to provide treatment that holds out no hope of cure, remission, palliation, or anything other than possibly a relatively short period of biological life. It does not seem right that patients, even dying patients, should have the power to command their physicians to perform any treatment that holds even a faint promise of longer biological life. But then, it also does not seem quite right that physicians should be able to deny a patient those moments the patient may deem to be of great value.

There is no "quick fix" solution to this problem, but certain principles should be considered when trying to work it out. First, it is an open question whether patients who say "do everything" literally mean what they are saying. Patients who say "do everything" or "I want my life to be prolonged to the greatest extent possible without regard to my condition, the chances I have for recovery, or the cost of the procedures" may not truly understand what they may be getting into. Second, clinicians have no legal or ethical obligation to perform useless treatment, even if the patient requests or demands it. But what does "useless" mean in this context? It must have something to do with the teleology of medicine itself: curing, healing, relieving pain, alleviating disability or dysfunction. The patient's will alone surely cannot render a treatment "useful." Third, clinicians should be wary about promising that "everything will be done" when they may be unable or unwilling to comply for reasons ranging from the ethical to the financial.

In summary, because of the nature of AIDS as a progressive and incurable disease and of the demographics of the individuals who most often suffer from it, a patient's advance directives about the course of his or her medical care can be crucial to caring for that patient as an individual and to making the best clinical decisions.

## NOTES

1. B. Lo and R. S. Steinbrook. Deciding whether to resuscitate. *Archives of Internal Medicine* 143 (1983):1561–63.

2. J. F. Murray et al. Pulmonary complications of the acquired immunodeficiency syndrome: Report of a National Heart, Lung, and Blood Institute workshop. *New England Journal of Medicine* 310 (1984):1682–88.

3. *Bouvia* v. *Superior Court*, 179 Cal. App. 3d 1127 (1986).

4. L. Nelson. The law, professional responsibility, and decisions to forego treatment. *QRB* 12 (1986):8–15.

5. R. Steinbrook et al. Preferences of homosexual men with AIDS for life-sustaining treatment. *New England Journal of Medicine* 314 (1986):457–60.

6. Nelson, The law.

7. Calif. Civil Code S2430 et seq. (West 1986).

8. Steinbrook et al., Preferences of homosexual men.

9. Ibid.

10. Calif. Civil Code S2430.

11. *In the matter of Conroy*, 486 A. 2d 1209 (NJ 1985) and *In the matter of Saunders*, 492 N.Y.S. 2d 510 (Su. Ct. 1985).

# 11 AIDS AND THE ALLOCATION OF INTENSIVE CARE UNIT BEDS

*Ray E. Moseley*

The AIDS epidemic forces us to come to grips with a number of different problems in the allocation of health care resources. On the national level we must decide how much is to be spent on basic research, on education, and on epidemiological studies. On the regional level decisions must be made about whether to designate specific hospitals as AIDS treatment centers, how best to fund them, and how to support care for indigent AIDS patients. On the institutional level, decisions about AIDS focus on the allocation of available hospital beds and health care personnel. It is on this level that I will confine my comments. In particular, I shall examine some institutional policies on the use of relatively scarce intensive care facilities for AIDS patients. My analysis rests on four assumptions about this issue:

1. We do, in fact, allocate intensive care unit (ICU) space, both informally and formally.[1]
2. There will be few, if any, additional health care dollars available now or in the near future for expansion of ICU facilities.
3. The number of AIDS cases and the need for their treatment will continue to increase significantly over the next several years and will put additional burdens on intensive care facilities.[2]
4. A significant number of AIDS patients will be in an ICU setting at some point during the course of their illness.[3]

In the context of these assumptions, I will discuss three kinds of criteria that have been used to allocate ICU beds for AIDS patients: "social worth," "economic costs," and "benefit to the patient." These methods of allocating ICU beds were identified in a national survey directed to ICU directors of major hospitals.[4] These three allocation methods all raise general issues about the fair use of ICU resources and particular questions about whether it is ever appropriate to exclude AIDS patients from the ICU setting. I argue that benefit to the patient is the only allocation criterion acceptable from a moral point of view. Since even the application of this criterion has serious potential for abuse, institutions should establish policy guidelines governing the allocation of ICU beds that include formal procedures to guide decision making.

## SOCIAL WORTH CRITERIA

Although it is difficult to document, there is much anecdotal evidence that AIDS patients have been excluded from ICU beds solely because of the patient's perceived *social worth*.[5] Much of this discrimination probably results from unjustified homophobia.[6] However, if sheer prejudice could be avoided, one might argue that social worth could be one legitimate way by which to allocate health care resources. For example, during disasters we justify treating health professionals and fire fighters first because of the social utility of having them back in action to help the rest of us. In the absence of this sort of public emergency, however, attempts to use this "triage" model hinges on being able to fairly define and evaluate social worth.

Two sorts of problems plague this approach, which render it virtually useless—from a moral point of view—for making ICU allocation decisions. First, in the absence of public calamity it is very difficult to decide how to measure social worth. For example, it is simply not clear how to weigh the contributions of an artist against those of a banker, physician, or journalist. Second, the experience with this approach indicates that it is very difficult to apply measures of social worth fairly, even when they can be justified.[7] Even when overt prejudice is avoided, the individuals who make the allocation decisions tend to direct resources to the patients who most resemble them physically and socioeconomically.

## COSTS OF CARE

Another reason sometimes cited by ICU coordinators to exclude AIDS patients from an intensive care setting is that AIDS patients simply *cost* too much.[8] For example, the average lifetime cost per AIDS patient from diagnosis to death ranges from $50,000 to $150,000 based on an average survival time of 18 months.[9] The majority of these costs reflect the duration of the hospital stay, with a significant percentage attributed to ICU costs.[10] It is argued that as a discreet class of patients, AIDS patients consume so many of the available health care dollars, especially if treated in intensive care facilities, that society simply cannot afford to provide them with maximal care. This argument takes on added weight with the projected increase in the number of AIDS patients. Following this argument, it could be concluded that the resources needed to provide intensive care to all AIDS patients who require it will be simply unavailable.

It should be recognized that our society already does make decisions about how to allocate research and treatment resources by disease categories. We have lobbying groups for cancer, diabetes, heart disease, muscular dystrophy, etc. Thus, at the level of macroallocation decisions one might argue that the economic burden of financing AIDS intensive care is not worth the projected benefit. To successfully hold this position one must measure and compare the predicted benefits of ICU care for all disease categories for which it might be considered.

The difficulty here is that this line of argument wrongly concludes that AIDS patients are easily grouped into a class of individuals who use a great deal of economic resources and whose prognoses are all similar. In reality, the symptoms and clinical course of AIDS vary a great deal among patients. Some AIDS patients (and it is not clear how well we can identify which ones) may greatly benefit by ICU care in terms of either increased length of survival or a temporarily improved quality of life. Other diseases have similarly poor prognoses and erratic courses (such as serious heart or respiratory disease) and seem no different in any relevant way, either in cost of treatment or quality of life, from that of AIDS. It would clearly be unjust to single out AIDS patients as a class unless the same cost-benefit criteria were applied across the board to all other diseases. It is far from clear that AIDS patients would be excluded from ICU care if these comparative analyses were made.

## BENEFIT TO THE PATIENT

The most obvious way to decide which patients should be in an ICU is by looking at whether ICU care, as opposed to treatment in a general hospital setting, would change the outcome for the patient, either by *likelihood* or *length* of survival or in *quality* of survival. In other words, will the patient *benefit* from ICU care? For some patients ICU care is no different, in terms of these categories of benefit, than care in a regular ward. For some patients, treatment in an ICU might enhance biological survival but quality of life might be very poor or nonexistent (as with the patient in a permanent coma). In these cases it is clear that the ICU is an inappropriate setting. A balance of quality of life and length and likelihood of survival must be maintained. If either quality or length of life or likelihood of survival is very low, ICU care may be inappropriate unless there is a greater and corresponding benefit in another area.

ICU care is likely to make some positive difference for many seriously ill patients, including AIDS patients. However, it is unfortunately impossible to put all patients who might benefit in any conceivable way, however small, into an ICU. Thus, it is necessary to decide what level and type of possible benefit to the patient justifies the use of ICU facilities.

In addressing the problem of determining an appropriate level of benefit that must be expected in order to place a patient in an ICU (given its size), it is helpful to remember the general purpose of the intensive, expensive, high-tech, ICU setting, where highly trained personnel are constantly monitoring the patient. The basic purpose is to bring these medical resources to a patient who needs to be rescued from a critical medical episode, that is, a patient whose needs and potential for recovery are both high. Thus, the level of potential benefit expected for a particular patient in order to gain ICU admission may very well be higher than the "any possible benefit" standard.

## THE ROLE OF A "TERMINAL" DIAGNOSIS

One common way of selecting patients as appropriate for ICU admission (that is, as likely to benefit at an acceptable level, given the cost) is by deciding which ones are "terminally" ill. The reasoning is that if a patient is going to die from the disease no matter how intensive the intervention, then the possibility of short-term gain is not worth the extreme cost or effort. The obvious implication of this guideline for ICU AIDS policies would be that, to the extent that AIDS is defined as a terminal illness, AIDS patients would not be appropriate candidates for the ICU.

Of course, the difficulty with this guideline is determining what counts as a "terminal" illness. There seem to be at least three different ways in which terminal illness is understood. It is either defined in terms of (1) imminent death (usually within 48 hours) or (2) short-term survival (usually up to six months) or it is defined by the fact that (3) the disease will *eventually* be fatal.

AIDS is not a stereotypical "terminal" illness under the first two definitions, but it does fit the third: AIDS appears to be uniformly fatal. However, the length of survival of AIDS patients after their first infection or the first onset of symptoms varies a great deal. AIDS patients may survive several years or die within months of the appearance of the first symptoms. The average survival from onset of first symptoms is *about eighteen months*.[11] Thus, if an ICU policy restricts AIDS patients' access because they are considered "terminal," only the third meaning of "terminal" must be operative. If this is the case, however, *all* patients who are being considered for the ICU must pass the test of this definition. One meaning of "terminal" cannot be used when considering AIDS patients and another meaning of the term used when considering other patients for ICU placement. It should be noted, however, that current practice in most ICUs indicates that many patients who will eventually die from their disease are routinely admitted.[12]

Second, it is not uncommon for the "terminal" AIDS patient to go through a number of crises during the course of the illness. Hospitalization in intensive care settings sometimes enables the patient to recover from the immediate crisis and return home.[13] For example, about half of AIDS patients enter the hospital with pneumocystis pneumonia. Although the presence of pneumocystis pneumonia (even when controlled by aggressive treatment) signals almost certain death within a year, this disease can often be effectively treated in the short run, and the patient may recover to the point of independent function. In these cases ICU care offers significant benefit in terms of the quality of the AIDS patient's survival as well as a moderate extension of the patient's life expectancy.

Confusion over the meaning of "terminal" may be a sufficient reason why its use should be avoided in policies governing ICU resource allocations. Currently, 16 percent of hospitals report that they do not accept AIDS patients in their ICU because the patients are "terminally ill."[14] Clearly, if the term is used in defining an ICU admitting policy, a meaning should be specified to avoid the unjust situation of applying the term differently in cases where there are no ethically or medically relevant differences.

But which definition of "terminal" *should* be used, granting the term *will* be used, in assessing appropriateness of ICU care? The first sense seems preferable, since many diseases that are uniformly fatal may, with ICU intervention, still allow an acceptable quality of life for at least some of the time before the person's death. Although it should be noted that the arbitrariness of defining what counts as "imminent" death continues to be a problem, it is at least less ambiguous than "terminal" when applied to fatal, irreversible illnesses. However, if this definition of "terminal" is used, it cannot be employed to describe AIDS patients or as a reason to restrict AIDS patients from ICUs.

## CONCLUSION

It would seem entirely acceptable to treat particular AIDS patients in ICUs, especially as our ability to determine which AIDS patients will benefit from intensive care increases. We should not exclude AIDS patients from ICU care because (1) they have little social worth (as determined by some individuals); (2) as a class they use too many of our economic resources; or (3) they cannot benefit from ICU care. However, one should not conclude from these arguments that health care institutions are obligated to treat every AIDS patient in an ICU. Rather, I conclude that institutions should not refuse to treat AIDS patients in ICUs on those three grounds. Unfortunately, discrimination against AIDS patients is already accepted by much of the population on social grounds. There is real danger that allocation decisions based on economic criteria may mask this discrimination against AIDS patients.

Of course, macroeconomic decisions about the funding of ICU care may still exclude AIDS patients from ICUs, even where admittance criteria are based on acceptable minimum levels of possible benefit to patients. The level of "possible benefit" that a patient must meet to be admitted to an ICU will always vary depending on available beds. Given a situation of unlimited economic resources, including ICU beds and trained health care personnel, the problem of allocation would not be serious. In this situation we might set the admittance criteria such that "any possible benefit" to a patient from ICU care would be adequate. However, a standard more stringent than "any possible benefit" must be adopted given current and projected macroeconomic constraints. Similarly, the prospect of any great increase in number of ICU beds to handle the possibly 1 million or more currently infected persons when they become symptomatic is dim. Up to this point in the epidemic ICU space has been generally available except in some high-incidence areas.[15] The "any possible benefit" standard of access to an ICU will be raised and use of the level of "possible benefit" as an admitting criterion will steadily increase as the number of patients increases. Thus we may come to a point where no AIDS patient could possibly benefit to the degree required to gain access to the ICU. As long as this standard of benefit is applied equally to *all* patients a charge of unjust restriction of AIDS patients from ICUs is not appropriate *even though* no AIDS patients would, in fact, be admitted to the ICU. This continuing shift of the "benefit" measure requires institutions to be constantly monitoring their intensive care situation and updating their admittance policies and procedures as pressures on the ICUs increase. Because criteria will vary as pressure on the ICUs increases, policymakers must be vigilant to avoid the danger of unfairly singling out AIDS patients for denial of ICU access.

The predicted increase in the number of AIDS patients mandates that each institution work toward policy guidelines about ICU admission procedures. It is likely that the increase in patients will shortly outstrip the number of available ICU beds. Our institutional policies should reflect a belief that we must allocate ICU space on the basis of the *benefit* to patients. Further, the allocation of ICU space should not be done on an informal basis in the absence of peer and administrative review. The proven dangers of unfair discrimination are simply too great.

# NOTES

1. H. T. Engelhart, Jr., and M. Rie. Intensive care units, scarce resources, and conflicting principles of justice. *Journal of the American Medical Association* 255 (1986):1159–64 and M. J. Strauss et al. Rationing of intensive care unit services. *Journal of the American Medical Association* 255 (1986):1143–46.

2. R. Steinbrook et al. Ethical dilemmas in caring for patients with the acquired immunodeficiency syndrome. *Annals of Internal Medicine* 103 (1985):787.

3. Ibid., 788.

4. R. Moseley. AIDS and ICU allocation: A survey of ICU directors. University of Florida, 1986–87. Manuscript, Medical Humanities Program, Department of Family and Community Medicine, J. Hillis Miller Medical Center, Gainesville, Fla.

5. Ibid.

6. A. Zuger. Professional responsibilities in the AIDS generation. *Hastings Center Report* 17 (June 1987):18. T. Kalman, C. M. Kalman, and C. J. Douglas. Homophobia among physicians and nurses: An empirical study. Abstract 225, Second International Conference on AIDS. Paris, France, June 23–25, 1986.

7. J. Childress. Who shall live when not all can live? *Soundings* 53 (Winter 1970):339–55.

8. Moseley, AIDS and ICU.

9. Institute of Medicine and National Academy of Sciences (IMNAS). *Confronting AIDS: Directions for Public Health, Health Care and Research.* Washington, D.C.: National Academy Press, 1986, p. 156.

10. E. J. Graves and M. Moien. Hospitalization for AIDS, United States 1984–85. *American Journal of Public Health* 77 (1987):729–30. A. M. Hardy et al. The economic impact of the first 10,000 cases of acquired immunodeficiency syndrome in the United States. *Journal of the American Medical Association* 255 (1986): 210.

11. IMNAS, *Confronting AIDS*, 156.

12. Moseley, AIDS and ICU.

13. Steinbrook et al., Ethical dilemmas, 788.

14. Moseley, AIDS and ICU.

15. Steinbrook et al., Ethical dilemmas, 788.

# 12 AIDS AND THE DUTY TO INFORM OTHERS
## William J. Winslade

Public alarm and professional concern in response to the AIDS epidemic have generated numerous proposals to decrease the spread of AIDS. These include quarantine or identification of persons with or known to be at risk for AIDS, voluntary testing of persons in high-risk groups, or even involuntary mass screening of the general population. However, stigma, rupturing of personal relationships, and discrimination are difficult to avoid for those individuals who are identified as having AIDS or the HIV antibody. This provides a powerful motive not to disclose relevant facts about oneself with respect to AIDS, even when contemplating conduct that exposes others to the risk of contracting a potentially fatal illness. Much debate, both reasonable and irresponsible, has taken place as policymakers consider alternative legal and public approaches to the problem. In response to extreme and sometimes hysterical reactions, it is important to examine carefully and calmly the *moral* rights and responsibilities of those with or known to be at risk for AIDS and the moral duties of the professionals who treat them.

In this essay I examine two specific moral issues faced by individuals who have AIDS or carry the antibody to the AIDS virus, or are known to be at risk for AIDS[1] (hereafter collectively called "risk carriers") and their health care providers. Do risk carriers or their providers have a duty to *inform* others who have been or may be exposed to the risk of AIDS? Do risk carriers or their providers have a duty not to expose others to the possibility of infection?

I argue that risk carriers do have a compelling moral responsibility not to expose others unknowingly to the risk of a fatal infectious disease. It is also clear that risk carriers have a moral duty to inform others who may be or may have been at risk for AIDS because of contact with the risk carrier. Not only does an appropriate disclosure directly respect the autonomy and right of others to know, but it also indirectly helps to protect third parties who might otherwise unknowingly be exposed to a risk of infection. However, the moral duty to disclose extends only to those actually placed at risk. Risk carriers are still entitled to protect their privacy. Disclosure of one's status as a risk carrier to persons not exposed to the risk of infection, while morally permissible, is not obligatory.

The moral duties of the health care professional who treats the risk carrier are similar. The professional has a duty to preserve the privacy of the risk carrier as well as to prevent the harm to others that can be directly caused by the patient or client. Sometimes this can be accomplished by the professional's persuading the patient or client to make the necessary disclosure or take appropriate precautions against exposing others to the the risks of infection. It may, in some circumstances, be necessary to disclose otherwise private or confidential information to third parties, or it may be sufficient to inform threatened third parties in a way that does not identify a particular patient or client or disclose otherwise confidential information. The professional must negotiate a narrow path between fidelity to patients and clients and responsibility to protect persons placed at risk of harm by the professional's patient or client.

In this chapter I take for granted the assumption that one has moral duties to prevent harm to and respect the autonomy of others. Similarly, I assume that informing others that they have been or may be exposed to the risk of AIDS is one important way to respect autonomy and prevent harm. Both common morality and law endorse respect for personal autonomy and harm prevention; much ethical theory attempts to justify these values. Finally, I do not try to justify the dual moral duties of professionals to their patients or clients as well as to third parties. My aim is to apply these well-established moral duties to situations related to AIDS.

To illustrate the way in which moral duties to others arise in the context of the AIDS epidemic, I will consider the moral implications of the lawsuit filed against the Rock Hudson estate and other defendants. I will also draw upon the analogy to a well-known case concerning the duties to third parties of psychotherapists with dangerous patients. Let me stress that in referring to these legal cases, my aim is to illuminate the nature and scope of *moral* duties. I do not discuss the enforcement of morality or the closely related legal issues concerning liability for failure to protect third parties from harm. A clearer understanding of underlying moral considerations, however, will help illuminate issues concerning moral sanctions or legal liability. Nor does my analysis address the public health or political problems that are, of course, of enormous concern. But clarity about the moral issues may help to explain as well as justify action taken in these other contexts.

## THE ROCK HUDSON CASE

On November 27, 1985, a lawsuit was filed by Mark Christian against Rock Hudson's estate, the administrator of his estate, Hudson's secretary, and his physicians.[2] The complaint is based in part upon the alleged failure of Hudson and others to inform Christian that Hudson had AIDS. It is asserted that Hudson violated a fiduciary duty, derived from the love relationship between Hudson and Christian, to inform Christian that Hudson had AIDS, had exposed Christian to the risk of contracting AIDS, and that further sexual contact had increased the risk. It is also claimed in the complaint that the other defendants conspired to conceal and did conceal information about Hudson's condition from Christian.

Whatever may be the results of the lawsuit, it does raise important moral questions. What moral duties, if any, does a person who is a risk carrier for AIDS have toward past, present, and future sexual partners? Similar questions could be raised about the moral duties of an IV drug user with or at risk for AIDS who shares needles with others. What duties arise to inform or protect others from risk?

If Hudson did not inform Christian of his prior exposure, and hence his potential infectiousness, then Hudson violated a general moral duty to others as well as a specific duty to Christian. Once Hudson had told Christian of the risk of harm, Christian could then choose whether to take further risks with Hudson. By giving Christian this information and an opportunity to choose, Hudson would have respected Christian as an autonomous person; by failing to inform Christian, Hudson would have violated a duty not only to Christian, but also to other parties (Christian's future sexual partners) and prevented Christian from informing other persons he may have already infected. Failure to inform Christian would have also violated Hudson's duty to respect Christian's autonomy regarding further sexual contact with Hudson and prevented Christian from informing his future sexual contacts so that Christian could respect their autonomy.

Thus, once Hudson learned that he had AIDS, he incurred a moral duty to inform Christian of his past exposure to the risk of infection and potential additional risk in the future. Even if Hudson had decided to discontinue sexual relations with Christian after diagnosis of AIDS, he still would have had a duty to inform Christian of the prior exposure. Although Christian could not then do anything about the possibility that he was infected, he, in turn, could inform others of possible past exposure and forbear from exposing still others to the risk of infection.

It has been reported that Hudson sent anonymous letters to his previous sexual partners to inform them they may have been exposed to the AIDS virus. At first glance this may seem an insufficient response to those at risk. How do they know, for instance, that this letter is anything more than a cruel fraud? But it does put the recipients of the letter on notice; it might, for example, motivate a recipient to be tested for the antibody to the AIDS virus, to abstain from unsafe sex, or to seek counseling. Assuming that Hudson discontinued sexual liaisons with persons to whom an anonymous letter was sent, it is the exposure rather than the risk carrier's identity that is crucial. Syphilis and gonorrhea contact tracing by public health officials does not use names. Admittedly, an anonymous letter has less authority than an official notification, but the recipients may already realize that they are in a high-risk group. The letter discloses the possibility of exposure and to that extent recognizes their right to exercise options, including that of not exposing others. Thus an anonymous letter goes part of the way toward fulfilling the moral duties to inform others directly and to prevent harm to still others by advising the recipients of their potentially infectious condition. The disclosure of such information is an essential step in an effort to break the epidemic chain of transmission.

Thus far I have considered the moral duties of persons, like Rock Hudson, with a clear diagnosis of AIDS. Do persons who have had a positive test for the antibody to the AIDS virus or individuals known to be at risk for AIDS (for example, an IV drug user who has not been tested but has shared a needle with someone known to have AIDS) have a duty to disclose their status or protect others from the risk of exposure? It seems obvious that every risk carrier has a duty to inform past sexual contacts or needle sharers, though there are practical limits on how complete the notification can be. Similarly, disclosure to current contacts is obligatory in order to give such persons the opportunity to make their own decisions about risk taking. However, it could be argued that persons who are seropositive or known to be at risk could fulfill their moral duty to *future* contacts by avoiding unsafe sex, needle sharing, blood giving, or other kinds of behavior known to expose others to risks. Is disclosure of a risk carrier's status morally required if the likelihood of exposing others is negligible?

I believe that the duty to *disclose* is closely tied to the duty *not to expose* others to the risk of infection with a probably fatal disease. If one seeks to have a contact with another that will expose the other to risks, then disclosure is morally mandatory. If the other is not exposed to the risk of infection then disclosure is not required to prevent harm. Does respect for others' autonomy require disclosure of one's status apart from actual risk of exposure? It could be argued that disclosure of one's status is required to permit others to choose whether to continue even nonrisky associations. However, such disclosure undermines the privacy and autonomy of those who reveal their status. It is not wrong to disclose, but it is not obligatory to do so.

This analysis of the Rock Hudson case suggests that definite moral duties fall on AIDS risk carriers. In order to respect Christian's autonomy, Hudson had a moral duty to give Christian the information necessary to makes choices concerning future sexual liaisons with Hudson. And Hudson had a moral duty to inform Christian so that the latter could avoid exposing others to the risk of harm. Thus a key benefit of disclosure is to prevent an unknowing continuation in the chain of transmission. What about Hudson's physicians? Do they have similar duties of disclosure about Hudson's condition? To gain some perspective on their duties, let us first consider the *Tarasoff* case.

## THE *TARASOFF* CASE

The well-known *Tarasoff* case concerned the legal duties of psychotherapists in California who treat patients who are dangerous to others. The California Supreme Court formulated a legal rule derived from this case as follows:

When a therapist determines, or pursuant to the standards of his profession should determine, that his patient presents a serious danger of violence to another, he incurs an obligation to use reasonable care to protect the intended victim against such danger.[3]

Quite apart from the legal arguments for such a rule, it is easy to see that one moral underpinning of the rule is the duty to prevent harm to others. One could argue that the *Tarasoff* rule also appeals to a principle of paternalism: It enjoins the therapist not merely to warn the victim, out of respect for autonomy, but to go further; the therapist should take reasonable steps to *protect* the threatened third party from harm. Notwithstanding the duty of therapists to protect their patient's privacy, they have a duty to prevent harm to threatened third parties. Therapists have this duty because they are in a special position to know (or should know) the risk, cannot rely on the violent patient to restrain him- or herself or warn the victim, and are imbued with the authority and status that make a disclosure of risk credible.

The *Tarasoff* rule has provoked a decade of debate about its potentially chilling effect on psychotherapy, its difficulty to apply, and its violation of patient privacy.[4] But most observers do not deny, in at least some cases, that the potential harm to others overrides the other values listed just above. The serious threat of violence is the principal reason why the duty to protect a threatened third party overrides the other values. The law follows morality standards by endorsing the significance of preventing harm to others even though other duties to one's patient—such as respecting confidentiality—may be subordinated.

When the *Tarasoff* rule requires the therapist to warn the victim or notify the police or do whatever is reasonable to protect the threatened victim, it implicitly recognizes the importance of the victim's autonomy. Once officially put on notice the potential victim can then choose whether or not to associate with the potentially dangerous patient. That the *Tarasoff* rule may require more than a warning puts a paternalistic nuance on the legal rule, but in some cases a warning that respects the potential victim's autonomy may be sufficient.

The duties created by the *Tarasoff* rule are imposed directly on the therapist. This is no doubt in part based on the assumption that a person suffering from a mental disorder may not be willing or fully able to control his or her conduct. But the imposition of a duty on the therapist does not negate the patient's duty to commit no harm and to respect the autonomy of the potential victim.

## COMPARING THE HUDSON AND *TARASOFF* CASES

It is helpful to clarify further moral rights and responsibilities in AIDS cases by examining the similarities and differences between the Rock Hudson and the *Tarasoff* cases. First, both cases involved potentially serious harm even though the manner in which the risk of harm was created differed. In the *Tarasoff* situation the patient threatened to kill and eventually did kill his victim. In Rock Hudson's case sexual contact allegedly exposed Mark Christian to the risk of contracting a potentially lethal disease. Thus, each victim was exposed to a risk of death. Second, the dangerous patient and the risk carrier may both be a direct cause of harm. In fact in the *Tarasoff* opinion the California Supreme Court drew an analogy between diagnosing an infectious disease and diagnosing dangerousness. Just as the physician who makes a diagnosis of an infectious illness incurs duties to third parties, so also does a psychotherapist who makes a "diagnosis" of dangerousness. I am merely carrying the argument one step further. The duties of the physician or psychotherapist who *knows* the diagnosis of potential infectiousness of the patient or client, then, would have similar duties to third parties at risk. Third, if the dangerous patient is unable or unwilling to control the impulse to violence, the therapist incurs a duty to intervene. Similarly, if AIDS patients tell their physician or therapist that they are unable or unwilling to control impulses to engage in unsafe sex or if an AIDS patient suffered from a mental disorder that impaired competence or control of conduct, the therapist would have a duty to take reasonable steps to protect others from harm.

In many cases AIDS patients, unlike mentally ill or dangerous patients, are capable of warning or informing sexual partners of the risks. However, numerous pressures—fear of stigma, loss of love, shame, etc.—might cause a person with AIDS not to disclose relevant facts. In such cases physicians and psychotherapists do, I believe, incur a duty to try to persuade their reluctant patients to notify present and future sexual partners of the risks they are running. If their patient refuses to do so, physicians and therapists have a moral duty—based on the duty to prevent harm and to respect autonomy—to take reasonable steps to notify threatened sexual partners. I do not deny that there may be practical difficulties in carrying out such duties; however, the practical problems are rarely as difficult to overcome as those who resist carrying out their duties claim.

Therapists who can control the dangerous patient, for example, by convincing the person to enter a hospital voluntarily or by committing the patient without the latter's consent, may be able—at least for a time—to fulfill their duty without notifying a threatened victim or by disclosing otherwise confidential information. Similarly, to the extent that physicians or psychotherapists can convince their patients not to expose others to AIDS or can restrain them from doing so, the duty to others (at least with regard to future conduct) can be satisfied without warning others and hence disclosing otherwise confidential information. If the therapist is unable to persuade the patient to inform others who may have been exposed in the past, the professional does have a duty to convey relevant information to those who have been exposed. But in the absence of persuasion or power to control the patient's conduct, the therapist or physician has a duty to take other steps to prevent harm to others. What specific steps are required in each case may vary, but the duty to prevent harm and the proliferation of harm remains.

It has been reported that some AIDS patients suffer dementia due to neurological deterioration;[5] others may be depressed or even psychotic, though the latter is apparently uncommon. But those who deliberately expose other persons to the risk of a lethal disease may well be exhibiting pathological denial or personality disorders such as borderline personality. Such persons may superficially appear to be psychologically intact. Their conduct as risk carriers, however, may point to underlying mental impairment that puts their sexual conduct on a par with the potential for violence of dangerous patients.

This does not mean that AIDS patients who reject the duty to prevent harm or to respect the autonomy of others are necessarily mentally ill. It may only mean that such persons value their own needs or desires more highly than the rights of others. I have no illusion that moral duties automatically control conduct, especially where sexual conduct is at is-sue. But to the extent that sexual behavior (or needle sharing) is not subject to rational control by those who engage in it, such behavior increases the burden on physicians and therapists to discuss the behav-ior with their patients and, if necessary, to intervene.

Those duties limit the extent to which physicians and psychotherapists can be exclusively concerned with the interests of their patients. Physi-cians and therapists often prefer to concentrate their attention exclusively on the therapist-patient relationship. Ignoring the consequences of the sexual behavior of persons with AIDS is as morally myopic as disregard-ing the potential for violence of dangerous psychiatric patients. The thera-pist must walk a narrow path between loyalty to one's patient and duties to third parties.

Consider the following (actual) case: A psychotherapy patient had a former lover who had died from AIDS. The patient, partly out of fear, has not had a blood test for exposure to the AIDS virus. He does not want to be tested or to inform his sexual partners. One option he has with regard to future partners is celibacy or safe sex (however properly defined). But he has a duty to past sexual partners (with whom he had contact after exposure to the person who died from AIDS) to inform them of their risk. Each of them has a right to know, not only so that they can make future informed choices, but also so that they can duly warn others who may be at risk. Otherwise, the risk of spreading the epidemic increases and the duties to respect autonomy and protect others from the risk of harm are undermined.

If a person with AIDS refuses to inform and protect others, a physician or therapist has a duty to warn them. The professional's moral duty to others is to take the necessary steps to protect the threatened third par-ties from harm. This may require the professional to notify the person at risk, to prevent the risk carrier from exposing others to the risk of infec-tions, or to take other appropriate measures. The professional must ful-fill such duties while also attempting to fulfill duties to the patient-client to protect privacy and autonomy. Accordingly, the professional is not permitted, without client consent, to disclose otherwise confidential in-formation to third parties unless it is necessary to protect them. But if disclosure is necessary in order to protect third parties, it is not only permissible, but required.

## OBJECTIONS AND RESPONSES

It might be argued that whatever duties individuals with AIDS or at risk for AIDS have toward others, it is also incumbent upon those who engage in sexual relationships—if only because of self-interest—to ques-tion their sexual partners in order to discern the risks that may be involved. Those who do not assume reciprocal responsibilities to make inquiries, it could be argued, thereby assume the risk. Even if this pragmatic rule makes sense, it in no way relieves the risk carrier of the duty to inform others who may be vulnerable. I have not argued that the only moral duties fall on AIDS patients or their care providers. But I have argued that such duties are primary and central to an analysis of moral duties in the context of the risk of AIDS.

Another objection is that my analysis undermines the privacy and confidentiality rights of persons with AIDS. It is true that my position places limits on the scope of privacy and confidentiality, but they are not values that override the duty to prevent harm to others or respect the autonomy of others, especially when the harm is potentially a threat to others' lives and to public health and safety. So long as harm can be prevented and autonomy protected, one should strive also to preserve privacy and confidentiality.

Let me conclude by reiterating that AIDS is a terrible disease. Those who have it suffer enormously, and those at risk live in the shadow of death. It is unfortunate that risk carriers are burdened by the duty to disclose information that may subject them to stigma, discrimination, and the rupturing of personal relationships. Those who are the recipients of such information have a duty to respond with the empathy and moral respect that is owed to all persons who bear such a heavy burden. If those who are warned as well as others turn away from risk carriers, it diminishes us all as moral beings. If we morally demand so much from the afflicted, no less can be demanded from those fortunate enough to be forewarned about the risk of AIDS.

## NOTES

1. I include in this category only persons who because of their conduct or contacts have reason to believe they are risk carriers but who have not been conclusively tested.

2. *Christian* v. *Sheft et al.*, Complaint filed in the Superior Court of the State of California for the County of Los Angeles, Case No. C574153 (1985).

3. *Tarasoff* v. *Regents of the University of California*, 17C. 3d 425 (1976).

4. W. J. Winslade. Psychotherapeutic discretion and judicial decision: A case of enigmatic justice. In *The Law-Medicine Relationship: A Philosophical Exploration*, ed. S. F. Spicker, J. M. Healey, and H. T. Englehardt. Boston: Reidel, 1981, pp. 139–57. W. J. Winslade. After *Tarasoff*: Therapist liability and patient confidentiality. In *Psychotherapy and the Law*, ed. L. Everstine and D. S. Everstine. Orlando, FL: Grune & Stratton, 1986, pp. 207–21.

5. *Hospital & Community Psychiatry* 37 (1986):135–42.

# III   AIDS and the Public Health

# 13 RESTRICTIVE PUBLIC HEALTH MEASURES AND AIDS: AN ETHICAL ANALYSIS

*John C. Moskop*

Since its first identification in 1981, AIDS has emerged as a major threat to the public health in the United States. Intensive research efforts have not yet succeeded in producing an effective treatment or vaccine, and thus AIDS continues to spread and to kill virtually 100 percent of its victims. A Centers for Disease Control (CDC) report has estimated the costs in health care and lost income for the first 10,000 cases of AIDS at over $6 billion.[1] By 1991 the cumulative number of AIDS cases is projected to rise to 270,000, including 179,000 deaths.[2]

In the absence of a vaccine, public health efforts have focused on modification of personal behaviors likely to transmit infection. Thus, programs have disseminated information about AIDS and its modes of transmission in an attempt to discourage risky behaviors. Sharply reduced rates of sexually transmitted infections among gay men in San Francisco suggest that awareness of AIDS has caused major changes in their sexual behavior.[3] The use of newly developed screening tests on the nation's blood supply has also virtually eliminated transmission of HIV (human immunodeficiency virus) via blood transfusion, and heat treatment is similarly effective in protecting hemophiliacs from infection via clotting factor.

For AIDS, as for every public health problem, there exists a continuum of possible responses which range from encouraging voluntary behavioral changes to imposing rigid control over behavior. In the area of automobile seat belt use, for example, programs range from public education about the value of seat belts, to designing more comfortable seat belts, to

119

requiring the installation of seat belts in all vehicles, to making failure to use seat belts illegal, to requiring that autos be designed so that they cannot be driven unless the seat belts are in proper use. Efforts to encourage voluntary seat belt use, though least intrusive and objectionable to the general public, are also relatively ineffective.[4] Thus, many states have recently taken the more forceful step of making seat belt use mandatory.

As the AIDS epidemic continues to grow, many have questioned whether efforts to promote voluntary changes in high-risk behaviors alone can bring this "public health emergency" under control. Some have recommended additional measures that would limit personal privacy and individual freedom of action. Such measures are, however, problematic from a moral point of view because they require the subordination of one set of fundamental values—individual privacy and freedom—to another—public health and safety. Moreover, because 90 percent of current AIDS victims are gay men and intravenous drug abusers,[5] the major burden of invasive or coercive public health measures against AIDS would fall directly on them. Such measures could significantly worsen the serious problems of discrimination and stigmatization they already face.

In this chapter, I will examine several potentially invasive or coercive public health measures against AIDS. I will focus on the areas of screening, reporting, contact tracing, quarantining, and other measures that restrict personal freedom.

## A PRINCIPLE FOR PUBLIC HEALTH DECISION MAKING

Before moving on to the specific areas, however, let us reflect on what general principles should guide us in choosing restrictive public health measures. As noted above, we are faced with a conflict between individual freedom and privacy, on the one hand, and public health and welfare, on the other. Traditionally, U.S. society has given a special priority to individual freedom, restricting it only in extreme circumstances or for compelling reasons. One might, therefore, try to decide when a restrictive public health measure is justified by determining when a particular threat to the public health becomes "extreme" or "compelling." Perhaps this could be determined historically by studying past epidemics and the measures instituted to combat them, although, as Tauer points out, a number of past practices would surely be viewed as unethical today.[6]

I would like to suggest a weaker, quasi-utilitarian principle which, although insufficient alone to justify a public health initiative, should at least represent a necessary condition for acceptance. The principle is: Restrictive public health measures should be likely to prevent more suffering than they create through limitation of individual freedom. This principle gives no special priority to individual freedom, but simply balances the latter's value against that of prevention of suffering. Thus, though the principle may need to be supplemented by stronger means of protection of freedom, measures that cannot satisy this principle clearly show inadequate respect for individual freedom.

From the above principle follow some significant corollaries:

1. A clear and significant danger to the public health must exist in order to justify restrictive public health measures. We do not, for example, force people to take screening tests for athlete's foot or bar them from locker rooms if a test is positive.
2. Restrictive public health measures should be likely to be effective in alleviating the danger to the public health. For example, no one should be required to receive a vaccination against AIDS if there is no evidence that it will be effective in preventing the disease.
3. Public health measures should adopt the least restrictive alternative consistent with effectively diminishing the public health threat. For example, total isolation of persons with leprosy is unjustified if early detection and treatment can prevent transmission of the disease.

Keeping the above principle and its corollaries in mind, let us turn now to a consideration of specific AIDS control measures.

## VOLUNTARY HIV SCREENING

Screening tests for HIV infection were developed primarily for the purpose of providing protection against the transmission of the virus through blood transfusion. As the new screening tests were about to be released to blood banks early in 1985, many persons barred from donating blood because they were members of high-risk groups voiced a desire to find out their infection status. Under pressure from groups worried that high-risk individuals might donate blood in order to discover their antibody status, the federal government provided funding for alternative testing sites across the country to provide testing apart from blood donation.[7] Testing at these sites is purely voluntary, but significant disagreement exists over whether to provide the testing anonymously or to require that those tested identify themselves. Anonymous testing is the practice in several states but not in others, which require identification but promise confidentiality.

Strong arguments can be marshaled both for and against requiring identification of test subjects. Only if those tested are identified can they be contacted for follow-up. Such follow-up contacts are essential for providing new information, gathering epidemiological data, and, if appropriate, pursuing contact tracing. Many, however, fear that despite promises of confidentiality, test results may come to be used against those tested. This fear may prevent people at risk from seeking testing despite their desire to know more about their condition. For example, the explicitly homophobic attitudes of a number of public officials lend at least some support to gays' mistrust of government intentions toward them. Kenneth Wing has suggested that recent enforcement of laws against sodomy may be a harbinger of increasing legislative and judicial attacks on sexual privacy.[8] The U.S. Supreme Court has recently confirmed Wing's prediction by upholding a Georgia law that makes sodomy a crime; the Court ruled that the constitutional right of privacy does not apply to homosexual activity.[9] In the wake of this major setback for gay rights, public fear of AIDS may easily serve as a rallying point for further legal attacks on gays. For example, the Justice Department has ruled that some employers may legally fire an HIV carrier if their motive is to protect other workers.[10] No matter how it occurs, breach of confidentiality resulting in public dissemination of a positive test result is likely to have dire consequences for the person tested, including loss of job, loss of health insurance, and social stigmatization.

Returning to the "utilitarian principle" stated earlier, the question becomes: Which alternative (anonymity or identification) will result in the least suffering? Lack of information about the consequences of the two alternatives makes this a difficult question to answer. On the one hand, requiring identification of test subjects will provide important epidemiologic information about AIDS, but at the risk of exposing gays (and others) to discrimination or homophobic policies. On the other hand, anonymity will protect those wishing to be tested from the ill will of individuals or government, but at the risk of forgoing potentially important information about a deadly disease, information that might protect others. Tauer suggests that very strong guarantees of confidentiality could be provided by federal legislation on the model of the Drug Abuse Prevention, Treatment and Rehabilitation Act of 1972.[11] This law protects the confidentiality of drug-dependent persons even from criminal investigations. If Congress saw fit to pass similar legislation regarding AIDS, perhaps fears about revealing potentially damaging information would be reduced. Though the legislation may not prevent every breach of confidentiality, it may reduce the risk enough to obviate the need for a special system of anonymous reporting.

## MANDATORY SCREENING

Mandatory HIV screening has been initiated among some groups (army recruits,[12] prisoners[13]) and recommended for others (health care workers, dialysis patients).[14] Because requiring people to undergo testing represents a more significant limitation of individual freedom than requiring those requesting screening to identify themselves, mandatory screening should have a stronger justification. The major reason for mandatory screening programs is presumably that identification of infected individuals will permit more effective control of viral transmission. But, it may be asked, would mandatory screening enhance control of infection in a military or prison setting? If so, how? Furthermore, if control requires special treatment or segregation of infected individuals, will they not be subject to devastating consequences of stigmatization and discrimination? Soldiers and prisoners are generally powerless to resist institutional rules, but their availability and inability to resist testing do not constitute a justification for mandatory screening.

Glover and Starkeson have argued against mandatory screening of health care workers.[15] I believe their arguments can be generalized to oppose mandatory screening of most other low- *and* high-risk groups. In low-risk groups, the incidence of infection is so small that large numbers must be screened to detect a single case, and most positive ELISA (ensyme-linked immunosorbent assay) tests will be false positives, requiring additional confirmatory testing. Thus, both the high cost of testing and the risk of false positives make mandatory screening for low-risk groups inadvisable. Though testing of high-risk groups can be cost-effective, it depends on the prior identification of high-risk individuals. Because many such individuals may fear the potentially adverse consequences, they will resist identification and testing. Such testing will therefore require serious invasion of privacy and coercion and may have adverse consequences for those listed. It may thus prove to be less effective than voluntary programs. For all those reasons, mandatory screening of high-risk groups also seems unjustifiable. Finally, at least one political organization, Lyndon LaRouche's National Democratic Policy Committee, advocates mandatory screening of the entire population and quarantine of all infected individuals.[16] The committee's idea, presumably, is to achieve a "final solution" of the AIDS problem; the allusion to Nazism is deliberate, in view of the massive coercion their plan would require.

## MANDATORY REPORTING AND CONTACT TRACING

Closely related to screening is the public health interest in reporting and case surveillance. Early in its history, AIDS was added to a long list of infectious diseases whose diagnosis must be reported to public health authorities. The rationale for such reporting is clear—information about who has a disease and what risk factors they exhibit is essential for drawing conclusions about how the disease is transmitted and how transmission can be prevented. Reporting may also enable specific infection control measures to be taken, such as contact tracing. Thus, since the discovery of AIDS, the Centers for Disease Control (CDC) has been a major source of epidemiological information about the disease. Based on this rationale, however, if some information is good, more information is presumably better, and in fact, CDC recently recommended that states consider making HIV infection, as determined by antibody testing, a reportable condition.[17] Four states already require reporting of this condition.[18]

Such information will surely have epidemiological significance, but its value may be limited. Unlike AIDS patients, only a small, relatively self-selected group of infected individuals would be reported, namely, blood donors and those who voluntarily seek testing. Depending on the specificity of the tests used, some individuals may receive false positive results and be incorrectly reported as infected. Moreover, reporting test results to one or more outside agencies increases the risk of breach of confidentiality and subsequent adverse effects for reported individuals. Consider, for example, the fact that blood banks have agreed to report to the Department of Defense all active-duty military personnel who test positively for HIV antibodies.[19] Clearly, the potential for discrimination resulting from these reports is very significant. As in the case of non-anonymous screening, therefore, reporting of infected individuals may require very strong guarantees of confidentiality in order to minimize the potential harm to those tested.

Attempting to identify, notify, and treat the sexual contacts of diseased individuals is a common method for controlling sexually transmitted diseases, such as syphilis. Several authors have recently recommended contact tracing for controlling the heterosexual transmission of AIDS.[20] Tracing is thought to be cost-effective for heterosexual but not homosexual contacts because of the lower prevalence of the disease among heterosexuals and the presumed smaller number of sexual contacts. Contacts identified could, of course, be tested and counseled but, unlike syphilis patients, not cured. Another major difference between syphilis and AIDS is that syphilis does not confer the same stigma today as does AIDS. Notification of contacts severely compromises the confidentiality of a person diagnosed with AIDS or HIV infection, since contacts may have no compunctions about spreading this information within the community. Thus, though the benefits of contact tracing of heterosexuals may be substantial, including prevention of AIDS in children, they may not justify the loss of confidentiality and the subsequent risk of serious adverse consequences for the infected person. A possible compromise would be to urge infected individuals themselves to inform their sexual contacts, and to be sure testing and counseling are available for those contacts.

## QUARANTINES

The final area to be discussed is that of quarantines and other restrictions on freedom of movement and of association. Proposals in this area have taken several forms, including the closing of establishments in which high-risk behaviors occur; the barring of AIDS patients or infected persons from schools, jobs, or other environments; and the enforced detention or isolation of infected individuals. Despite the often drastic nature of these restrictions, some have received a great deal of attention and support; for example, millions followed AIDS patient Ryan White's struggle to return to a Kokomo, Indiana, public school.

There is, of course, moral and legal precedent for restricting personal freedom on public health grounds in both the control of infectious disease and the involuntary commitment of the mentally ill. I have argued that a restriction cannot be justified if it violates a "utilitarian principle." To evaluate the more drastic restrictions under consideration in this final section of the chapter, I will restate that principle and its three corollaries as a set of necessary conditions. In order for a measure to be justifiable it must satisfy at least these four conditions: (1) The person or place to be restricted poses a demonstrable threat to the public health; (2) the magnitude of the threat, as determined by its probability and severity, is greater than the harm to individual liberties threatened by the proposed restriction; (3) the proposed restriction *can* significantly lessen the threat; and (4) there is no less restrictive means available to accomplish the goal.

The controversy over San Francisco's bathhouses illustrates the difficulty of satisfying all these conditions. Closing the bathhouses probably satisfies the first three conditions, that is, it is an effective, but not unduly harsh, method of lessening the demonstrable threat of anonymous sexual contact with multiple partners. As Mills, Wofsy, and Mills point out, however, a less restrictive approach, in the form of regulations forbidding sexual contact in the baths and requiring the posting of educational and warning signs, was adopted by the San Francisco authorities.[21] The Health Department later ordered the closing of particular bathhouses found to be violating these regulations. The California Superior Court, however, did not uphold this order, but instead imposed further measures to inhibit sexual practices, such as requiring removal of cubicle doors and expulsion of patrons observed to be engaging in high-risk sexual activities. The problem with the court's measures, however, is that they, too, may prove to be ineffective. Thus, the least restrictive *effective* means of addressing this threat may in fact be closing the offending establishments.

Most proposals to bar AIDS patients or infected individuals from schools or jobs fail to satisfy one or both of the first two conditions mentioned above. For example, most schoolchildren with AIDS pose no demonstrable threat to classmates because (1) there is no evidence of viral spread through casual contact, (2) the chance of parenteral exposure to infected body fluids is minimal, and (3) even if such exposure should occur, the risk of transmission of a virus through a single limited exposure is very small.[22] Moreover, being barred from attending school is obviously a major disadvantage for these children. For similar reasons the CDC has recommended that health care workers who do not perform invasive procedures; personal service workers, such as barbers and manicurists; and food service workers not be restricted in their work on the basis of AIDS or HIV infection.[23]

Perhaps the most difficult problems in this area are raised by proposals to quarantine or incarcerate infectious individuals, especially those who continue to engage in high-risk activities. Such behaviors are known to transmit the virus, but how serious a threat each *particular* individual poses may be more difficult to demonstrate, since some AIDS patients and antibody positive individuals may not be infectious, some are not or are no longer sexually active, and some exposed individuals may never develop the disease. Moreover, if a threat can be demonstrated, will it always outweigh the severe hardship of enforced detention or isolation? Such individuals would presumably have to be detained as long as they are infectious, perhaps for the rest of their lives. Even if the threat is serious enough to justify detention, will the quarantine of a few individuals significantly lessen the threat, or will wholesale detention of infectious individuals be necessary? Since 1 million to 2 million people in the United States may already be infected with the virus, wholesale detention evokes the very negative image of internment of Japanese-Americans during World War II. To quarantine a few infectious persons may be counterproductive, since it could give members of high-risk groups a false sense of security about sexual and drug practices.[24] Finally, are there less restrictive alternatives to imprisonment or isolation? Mills, Wofsy, and Mills report a case of a Florida prostitute with AIDS who was confined to her home and ordered to wear a monitor that signaled the police if she strayed more than 200 feet from her telephone.[25] This is, perhaps, less restrictive than jailing, but it may not be effective. Was surveillance also necessary to insure that this person was not practicing prostitution at home? Though the reasons for wanting to protect others against persons who will not modify high-risk behaviors are clear, effective measures to accomplish this goal will need to be either highly restrictive or highly invasive. Any systematic attempt to implement such measures will pose difficult practical problems and be extremely costly.

Let us consider one last proposal which some may find less restrictive than quarantines. This proposal was offered with apparent seriousness by William F. Buckley in an op-ed article in the *New York Times*.[26] Buckley suggested that "everyone detected with AIDS should be tattooed on the upper forearm, to protect common-needle users, and on the buttocks, to prevent the victimization of other homosexuals." This proposal has obvious similarities to the infamous scarlet letter of Nathaniel Hawthorne's novel. Buckley, in fact, acknowledges the analogy with *The Scarlet Letter*, pointing out that the scarlet letter was designed to evoke public condemnation, while the AIDS tattoo is designed for private protection. The intentions may well differ in the two cases, but the consequences—shame, violation of bodily integrity, stigmatization, and discrimination—are likely to be quite similar.

To sum up, this paper has reviewed some of the more controversial public health measures proposed to control AIDS. Serious doubts can be raised about the justifiability of a number of these measures even on the basis of a utilitarian principle that does not give special priority to the protection of individual freedom. Under that principle, public health measures must satisfy at least the four conditions listed previously. I have argued that in combatting AIDS neither mandatory carrier screening, nor contact tracing, nor quarantines can fulfill these four conditions.

## NOTES

1. A. M. Hardy et al. The economic impact of the first 10,000 cases of acquired immunodeficiency syndrome in the United States. *Journal of the American Medical Association* 255 (1986):209–11.

2. D. M. Barnes. Grim projections for AIDS epidemic. *Science* 232 (1986): 1589–90.

3. J. W. Curran et al. The epidemiology of AIDS: Current status and future prospects. *Science* 229 (1985):1352–57.

4. L. S. Robertson et al. A controlled study of the effect of television messages on safety belt use. *American Journal of Public Health* 64 (1974):1071–80.

5. Centers for Disease Control. Update: Acquired immunodeficiency syndrome—United States. *Morbidity and Mortality Weekly Report* 35 (1986):17–21.

6. C. A. Tauer. The concept of discrimination and the treatment of people with AIDS. This volume, Chapter 14.

7. M. F. Silverman and D. B. Silverman. AIDS and the threat to public health. *Hastings Center Report* 15 (August 1985):S19–S22.

8. K. R. Wing. Constitutional protection of sexual privacy in the 1980s: What is big brother doing in the bedroom? *American Journal of Public Health* 76 (1986): 201–4.

9. *Bowers* v. *Hardwick*. *U.S. Law Week* 34 (1986):4919–29.

10. M. Clark. AIDS in the workplace. *Newsweek* (July 7, 1986):62–63.

11. Tauer, Concept of discrimination.

12. D. M. Barnes. Military statistics on AIDS in the U.S. *Science* 233 (1986):283.

13. K. Glasbrenner. Prisons confront dilemma of inmates with AIDS. *Journal of the American Medical Association* 255 (1986):2399–404.

14. S. A. Capps. Duke favors AIDS testing. *San Francisco Examiner* (April 9, 1986):A1, A10.

15. J. J. Glover and E. C. Starkeson. Health care professionals and the potential for the iatrogenic transmission of AIDS: An ethical analysis. This volume, Chapter 16.

16. Democracy's rusty weapon. *The New Republic* (April 14, 1986):7.

17. Centers for Disease Control. Additional recommendations to reduce sexual and drug abuse related transmission of human T-lymphotropic virus type III/lymphadenopathy associated virus. *Morbidity and Mortality Weekly Report* 35 (1986):152–55.

18. D. Fox. *AIDS: Implications for public policy.* Perspectives lecture. East Carolina University School of Medicine, Greenville, NC, March 24, 1986.

19. T. Beardsley. U.S. troops and AIDS. *Nature* 316 (1985):668.

20. D. F. Echenberg. A new strategy to prevent the spread of AIDS among heterosexuals. *Journal of the American Medical Association* 254 (1985):2129–30. M. Marmor, M. Lyden, and R. Grossman. Containing the AIDS epidemic. *Journal of the American Medical Association* 254 (1985):2059.

21. M. Mills, C. B. Wofsy, and J. Mills. The acquired immunodeficiency syndrome: Infection control and public health law. *New England Journal of Medicine* 314 (1986): 931–36.

22. Centers for Disease Control. Recommendations for preventing transmission of infection with human T-lymphotropic virus type III/lymphadenopathy associated virus in the workplace. *Morbidity and Mortality Weekly Report* 34 (1985): 681–86, 691–95.

23. Ibid.

24. Health Policy Committee, American College of Physicians and the Infectious Diseases Society of America. Acquired immunodeficiency syndrome. *Annals of Internal Medicine* 104 (1986):575–81.

25. Mills, Wofsy, and Mills, Acquired immunodeficiency syndrome.

26. W. F. Buckley, Jr. Crucial steps in combatting the AIDS epidemic: Identify all the carriers. *New York Times* (March 18, 1986):A27.

# 14 THE CONCEPT OF DISCRIMINATION AND THE TREATMENT OF PEOPLE WITH AIDS
## Carol A. Tauer

Our society attaches great moral and legal weight to the principle of equality of people, and our religious traditions support this commitment. As a consequence, we attempt to identify and root out violations of the principle of equality, or those acts and practices that are called discriminatory.

In the popular and political debate about AIDS, the concept of discrimination is widely invoked. Those who favor mandatory testing and reporting, government contact tracing, closing of gay bathhouses, perhaps even some form of quarantine or isolation claim that such requirements would not be discriminatory, but would merely implement traditional public health practices which have been used successfully against other contagious diseases.

On the other side of the debate are those who are concerned that the lives of possible AIDS virus carriers may be ruined through denial of housing, employment, and insurance, and that their right to privacy in conducting their personal lives will be violated. Denials of such basic needs and rights are characterized as discriminatory.

In this chapter I show that these positions reflect two substantially different concepts of equality and discrimination, and that even when the concepts are sorted out, the notion of discrimination has limited value as a tool for analyzing the ethical issues in the AIDS debate. After reorienting the discussion in terms of two other concepts, autonomy and paternalism, I conclude with a consideration of society's legitimate interests in establishing measures to control the spread of AIDS.

## TWO VIEWS OF DISCRIMINATION

Philosophical discussions of discrimination and equality usually begin with Aristotle's dictum that equals must be treated equally, but unequals unequally in proportion to their inequality. Since no two individuals are equal in all respects, the principle is interpreted to refer to equality in whatever characteristics are relevant to the treatment under consideration. Discrimination occurs when people who are equal in the relevant characteristics are treated unequally.

One might infer from this analysis that if two people are both carriers of communicable diseases, they should be treated equally with respect to restrictions on their freedom and activities. However, the category of "communicable disease" is clearly too broad as a measure of equality, since different communicable diseases vary enormously in the manner of their spread and in their seriousness. The task is to find comparisons between pairs of diseases which are so similar that equal treatment of carriers is medically justifiable. The principle of equality would then confirm that equal treatment of carriers is also ethically justifiable.

This line of reasoning illustrates one interpretation of equality and discrimination. According to this interpretation, in order to determine whether a practice is discriminatory, one looks at other relevantly similar cases to see how they have been treated. If we treat the new type of case as we treated them, we cannot be accused of discriminating.

When considering AIDS as one communicable disease, we might find it to be similar to one disease in one respect, to another in some other. In some ways it is like hepatitis B or syphilis or leprosy. Moreover, if we refer to an era when people were ignorant of the etiology and effective treatment of most diseases, then anything from smallpox to the Black Death might be invoked for purposes of comparison.

In the ethical debate referred to earlier, one side relies on a comparison of AIDS with other communicable diseases. Restrictive and coercive public health measures have been used to control the spread of many of these diseases. Thus such measures may be used equally for the control of AIDS, and no discrimination would be present.

The first difficulty in applying this approach is a pragmatic one: making sure that the other diseases really are similar to AIDS in crucial respects. While mandatory reporting and contact tracing may be effective in the case of syphilis, might that be because anyone who had contracted syphilis would surely want to know in order to be treated and cured with antibiotics? Extensive precautions against contagion are used with carriers of hepatitis B, but is not hepatitis B more easily communicated than AIDS? Identification of cases and other disease control efforts resulted in the worldwide elimination of smallpox, but such methods have not led to the eradication of any sexually transmitted disease.

Moreover, the pragmatic difficulty of making relevant comparisons is not the main reason for rejecting the first interpretation of equality. Simply because carriers of similar diseases were or are treated a certain way, it does not automatically follow that it is ethically right to treat carriers of a new disease in the same way. Perhaps none of the infected should have been treated in that way.

If we look at the history of contagious diseases that present analogies to AIDS, we find a multitude of examples in which treatment of carriers was ethically questionable. Particularly when ignorance and fear are rampant (as they are now with AIDS), measures that are excessive and ineffective are often employed. The history of leprosy (Hansen's disease) provides one such example, in which the stigma and segregation imposed on those with the disease ruined countless lives unnecessarily. It was not until 1985 that provision for the "apprehension, detention, treatment, and release of persons" with leprosy was removed from federal law.[1]

Joan Trauner, a historian of science, cites the common practice of blaming epidemic diseases on minority groups, for example, the Chinese in San Francisco. Because they were viewed as socially and morally inferior, they were repeatedly made into scapegoats. In 1876, the city health officer declared that the cause of a smallpox epidemic was the presence "of 30,000 (as a class) of unscrupulous, lying and treacherous Chinamen" who had little regard for the health of the nation's people.[2] In 1880, the Board of Health condemned Chinatown as a nuisance, and in the 1890s buildings suspected of being sources of disease were repeatedly destroyed. In 1899, the entire Chinese quarter of Honolulu was burned to the ground for the same reason.[3]

Another disease often connected to moral failure is syphilis. For centuries, it was commonly held that God inflicted this disease on the human race to punish and correct its moral excesses. In the words of a physician at the court of Louis XV: "the Veneral Disease was sent into the World by the Disposition of Providence, either to restrain . . . the unruly Passions of a Sensual Appetite, . . . or to correct the gratification of them."[4] The medical profession perpetuated this view into the twentieth century when, combined with racism, it led to acceptance of the Tuskegee Syphilis Study, one of the most monstrous abuses in human subjects research in our history. Doctors wrote about the constitution of black males, which inclined them to uncontrollable and excessive sexual desire, including the unnatural desire for white women.[5] Reputable medical journals contained passages like the following, written by Thomas Murrell in 1906:

So the scourge sweeps among them. Those that are treated are only half cured, . . . the effort to assimilate . . . driving their diseased minds until the results are criminal records. Perhaps here, in conjunction with tuberculosis, will be the end of the negro problem. Disease will accomplish what man cannot do.[6]

Apparently then, one need have no qualms about using such beings as guinea pigs, as the U.S. Public Health Service did from 1932 to 1972.[7]

Even those who have noncommunicable diseases or disabilities have often been victimized by society. At times, society's interest appears to be merely that of avoiding unpleasant or offensive experiences, as witness the collection of "ugly laws" passed by various local governments. Until 1974, for example, the Chicago Municipal Code included this statute:

No person who is diseased, maimed, or mutilated or in any way deformed so as to be an unsightly or disgusting object or improper person to be allowed in or on the public places of this city, shall therein or thereon expose himself to public view.[8]

While I have presented some extreme examples, they show how ignorance and fear, especially when combined with prejudice against a minority group, have led to treatment which one surely could not ethically invoke as a precedent. To treat analogous diseases or conditions similarly could not be an ethical expression of the principle of equality.

A second interpretation of discrimination attempts to identify specific content in the concept of equal treatment. According to this interpretation, there are certain fundamental respects in which everyone must be treated equally. These include the basic human rights to justice, to freedom (of speech, religion, movement, association), to equality of opportunity (in education, employment, housing), etc. Side two in our debate, which upholds the rights of AIDS victims, invokes this concept of equality. Violating basic rights is discrimination. An AIDS virus carrier may not be deprived of these rights even if carriers of similar diseases were.

This reasoning seems valid; yet few rights are absolute. A right whose exercise affects other people cannot be absolute. For example, while I may have a right to risk my own health, I do not have a right to cause risks to yours without your knowledge and consent.

It follows that there are circumstances in which persons in a high-risk group or situation for contracting the AIDS virus would be morally required to seek or accept testing and to allow those who are immediately affected to know the results of a confirmed positive antibody test. (Here I assume that the meaning of the test results would be fully explained to the parties involved so that it is not misunderstood. Note, however, that a moral obligation does not entail that there should be a legal requirement for testing, which is a separate issue.) Typical examples of such cases and situations are: (1) a man who has had homosexual contacts within the last eight years and who is now contemplating sexual involvement with a new partner; (2) a hospital patient in a high-risk group when a health care worker has been inadvertently stuck by a needle contaminated with the patient's blood;[9] (3) a person admitted to a treatment program where the AIDS virus could be transmitted, as in renal dialysis.

What about the case of a gay man who has either not been tested or has tested positive and who continues to engage in unsafe sex? While he may be causing risks to others as well as to himself, given comprehensive public education programs we may presume that those who engage in these activities with him are aware of the risks and choose to accept them. This presumption would not hold if his contacts could not be expected to be normally well informed, for example, if they were of impaired mental ability or were teenagers; nor would it hold if the man in question were dishonest about his health or risk status. But if everyone involved is knowledgeable and consents, then overriding his (or their) basic rights is not justified on the grounds of protecting the rights of other individuals.

In its emphasis on individual rights, this second interpretation of discrimination focuses on personal autonomy. While preferable to the first interpretation, it is also ethically limited. In balancing one person's rights against another's, it provides a two-dimensional perspective. The full picture is seen only in three-dimensional perspective, where the interests of society—the common good or general welfare—are considered.

Those who espouse the focus on individual autonomy that dominated health care ethics in the 1960s and 1970s might argue that society's interest in AIDS is limited to providing resources so that those who are immediately involved may use them as they deem most appropriate. In this view, society would allocate funding that the scientific and medical sectors could apply to research and clinical trials, that the high-risk communities could expend for the education of their members, and that health care institutions could use to subsidize the care of those who are ill. Under this model, society need not make decisions about the control of a disease that, as far as we know, is substantially limited to certain identifiable groups. It is up to individuals in those groups to choose the means of control they wish to employ.

Observers of health care ethics have noted, however, that the 1980s represent a broad shift away from the individualistic emphasis in ethics.[10] While it was necessary to focus on autonomy for a time in order to correct a paternalistic bias in medical treatment, autonomy is not the only value, nor is it a value that overrides or "trumps" all others. Since the bias has now swung toward individual autonomy, as Robert Veatch notes, we currently have the task of "recovering our sense of a moral community,"[11] one whose citizens have "some sense of a common good, shared ideas, common dreams, and a vision of the self that is part of a wider collectivity,"[12] to quote Daniel Callahan. An ethic that provides protection only for individual autonomy is an impoverished ethic, ignoring the rich traditions of both Western and Eastern philosophy in their perennial quest to identify the "common good" and the nature of a good society.

Unfortunately, many attempts to define the good society proceed by defining out of the moral community those whose mores or lifestyles are viewed as aberrant by the majority. Moreover, this type of exclusion tends to concentrate on sexual practices rather than on habits such as fairness, honesty, and trustworthiness. For example, top government officials can be caught in one falsehood after another without being disavowed by the "moral majority." I would note that society cannot expect the gay community to cooperate in seeking the general welfare unless gay people are fully recognized as members of the moral community.

As a moral community seeking a common good, society may have a variety of differing interests related to the spread of AIDS. I would like to mention three that I consider significant.

## AIDS AND THE COMMON GOOD

The first interest society may have is a paternalistic one, expressed thus: Just as we may legislate that motorists use seat belts and motorcyclists wear helmets "for their own good," so we may require that gay men do certain things that will decrease their risk of contracting the AIDS virus. Since individual behavioral changes are difficult to monitor, society may promote its purposes obliquely, say by closing or regulating gay bathhouses. So the argument would run.

The history of contagious disease control shows that our era is not unique in reacting against such paternalistic prescriptions. For example, in relation to inoculation for smallpox, a member of the British Parliament in 1906 denounced the policy then current because "the liberty of doing wrong was still left among the privileges of freeborn Englishmen."[13] A recent quotation from the *New York Native* sounds tame by comparison: "It may be more important to let people die in the pursuit of their own happiness than to limit personal freedom by regulating risk."[14]

As we have learned from recent discussions about the paternalism of the medical profession, the individual (unless mentally incompetent) is in the best position to know what serves his or her own interests. I may prefer a long life, you may prefer an exciting or an active one. Since paternalism cannot truly serve the individual good it is intended to promote, a purely paternalistic policy will not really further the common good either. In Veatch's words, "The case is overwhelming that autonomy takes moral precedence over paternalism."[15]

The second interest society may have regarding the spread of AIDS is related to distributive justice. In promoting the common good, society has the function of making decisions about the distribution of its resources. It is ethically imperative that common resources be distributed both fairly and prudently (that is, effectively). AIDS is a catastrophic illness with enormous costs. The Centers for Disease Control estimates that approximately $147,000 is expended for the hospital care of each patient with AIDS.[16] (This figure reflects the high cost of care in New York. In San Francisco, a viable program of community services provides for extensive home care, and the average cost per patient is considerably less.) The total cost of the first 10,000 cases of AIDS is estimated at more than $6.3 billion in hospital fees and lost income.[17]

Whatever the source of reimbursement for such costs, they ultimately come out of the pockets of fellow insurees and taxpayers. Society has a legitimate interest in seeing to it that this money is not spent needlessly and that the expenditure does not deprive those who are in need of other types of basic services. Thus society has a legitimate and critical interest in preventing the further spread of AIDS. While advocates of the priority of personal autonomy may validly argue against any *paternalistic* intrusion on freedom of choice, they cannot argue that society should take no interest in how its resources are expended. And it would be immoral to propose that society simply ignore the needs of the sick.

A third interest of society is the desire to have a community that is as disease-free as possible, especially with respect to communicable diseases. With the introduction of vaccines in the nineteenth century and of antibiotics in the twentieth, the hope emerged that one after another of the communicable diseases would be eradicated. This goal has been reached on a worldwide scale with smallpox, and at the national level with many diseases. The view of health as an international ideal is expressed by the World Health Organization in language that is both rhetorical and utilitarian:

The enjoyment of the highest attainable standard of health is one of the fundamental rights of every human being. . . . The health of all people is fundamental to the attainment of peace and security. . . . The achievement of any State in the promotion and protection of health is of value to all. Unequal development in different countries in the promotion of health and control of disease, especially communicable disease, is a common danger.[18]

The inability to control communicable disease is regarded as a societal failure with political implications.

It is true that although syphilis is curable, the number of cases has continued in epidemic proportions in this country.[19] It is also true that experts in epidemiology have classified the sexually transmitted diseases among those whose eradication can be virtually ruled out.[20] Yet, until an epidemic of a fatal sexually transmitted disease occurred, we had the sense that we were well on the road to the commonly accepted goal of eliminating life-threatening communicable diseases from our communities. With the onset of AIDS, the health goals that just ten years ago were believed to be within our grasp have slipped immeasurably far from us. It is understandable that society would experience some discouragement, frustration, and impatience at this turn of events. There is a sense of collective failure.

It is interesting to note that two differing views about the most effective approach to the control of AIDS have epidemiological parallels over the centuries.[21] One approach, the reporting of cases and tracing of contacts, is related to "contagionist" theories of disease, theories that existed before they were scientifically verifiable. As early as 1546, Girolamo Fracastoro attributed smallpox and measles to "specific seeds" (*seminaria*) that were communicated through contact or through intermediate agents.[22] Proponents of this theory, or "contagionists," advocated identification of the diseased, isolation of cases, and quarantine of suspected contacts. In fact, it was a carefully planned strategy of case-by-case reporting and contact identification that finally succeeded, in 1977, in eradicating smallpox worldwide, when more general efforts at educating and vaccinating had failed.[23]

The other approach to controlling AIDS, a massive educational campaign aimed at convincing people to change their behavior, is analogous to methods based on the historical view that diseases arise out of unhealthy environments and living conditions. Holders of this view, including the great Thomas Sydenham, were called "sanitarians," or simply "anticontagionists;" and for several centuries preceding this one, the controversy between them and the "contagionists" was lively and even bitter,[24] as is the analogous controversy today.

The provision and use of HIV antibody testing is probably essential to an effective application of either of the cited strategies for controlling AIDS. It is obvious that testing for possible carriers is essential if one wishes to use the method of locating, informing, and counseling contacts. But it can also be argued that testing is needed in relation to an educational effort. Behavioral changes are much more likely to be made if it is clear exactly who needs to make them. Two gay men in a monogamous relationship who have not been exposed to the virus need make no changes in their sexual practices because of fear of AIDS.

The gay community may be able to use alternate or additional mechanisms for controlling the spread of AIDS, but society has at its disposal basically these two approaches, with variations. In a situation that impinges as seriously on society's interests as this one does, it would seem wise to employ both approaches simultaneously. Yet they both have substantial social costs.

A massive educational program requires providing public information about sexual practices that some people find objectionable for religious or moral reasons and that others regard as offensive when presented in the public media. In addition, these practices may be against the law in some jurisdictions, as is intravenous drug use. However, information on "safe sex" or the need for clean drug needles is easily available to people who read newpapers or who have access to other print sources of current information. If this information is not provided in a wider variety of media (radio and TV spots, billboards, through schools, workplaces, and social service agencies), then essential health information is being provided in a discriminatory way. Those who are illiterate, of low socioeconomic status, or teenagers will not have access to facts they need to know.

The social costs of the other approach, a reporting and contact tracing program, do not fall solely on those who are at high risk for AIDS. Such a program has the potential for promoting distrust and animosity between segments of our citizenry. Suspicions are expressed in questions like these: Even though the names reported in connection with other venereal diseases have never been disclosed, might not this disease be different? If anonymous reporting of cases is permitted, why should the contacts of these cases be specified by name? And the keeping of lists in itself has a sinister connotation.

The potential for harm from a lapse in the confidentiality that is promised to people tested for AIDS antibodies is enormous. Measures for protecting this confidentiality must be proportionately strong and carry penalties for violations. Only action at the federal level can carry the weight needed to insure that individuals will be protected and public health programs given a chance to be effective.

A precedent for federal legislation protecting confidentiality is found in the Drug Abuse Prevention, Treatment, and Rehabilitation Act of 1972.[25] In order to encourage drug-dependent individuals to enter treatment programs, Congress undertook to guarantee the confidentiality of "identity, diagnosis, prognosis, or treatment" of participants in these programs. It is illegal to disclose such information, even in order to initiate or substantiate criminal charges. AIDS is a public health problem that merits equally vigorous action at the national level.

In addition, other mechanisms for preventing inadvertent or malicious violations of confidentiality should be creatively explored. Social scientists, for example, have developed clever ways of storing survey and informant data to keep it confidential. By encoding the data in complex ways and by distributing it among several locations, these researchers make it impossible for any one worker to put it all together or to link any data with any specific name. Even a subpoena can be avoided by such systems.[26]

Society has legitimate interests in stopping the spread of AIDS. It is clearly in the interests of everyone, particularly those in high-risk groups, that the disease be brought under control. If society does not undertake vigorous public health efforts, it could be accused of thus paraphrasing Murrell's comment on blacks and syphilis: "Perhaps here . . . will be the end of the [homosexual] problem. Disease will accomplish what man cannot do."[27]

In everyone's interest, we must stop the spread of AIDS. But we must be creative enough to find measures that will not do more harm than good. I have argued that the concept of discrimination has a limited value in this effort. Both of the interpretations of equality that might stand behind the concept would lead us to neglect society's obligations to distribute its resources fairly and promote the public health. Given the protections that the principle of individual liberty requires and the insights that the histories of other epidemics can provide, these societal obligations can justify a national program of AIDS education and confidential use of the AIDS antibody test.

## NOTES

1. 42 U.S.C. S 247e, before amendment of October 7, 1985.

2. J. B. Trauner. The Chinese as medical scapegoats in San Francisco, 1870–1905. *California History* 57 (1978):70–87.

3. Ibid, 73–77.

4. Quoted in S. Andreski. The syphilitic shock. *Encounter* 55 (1980):79.

5. A. M. Brandt. Racism and research. The case of the Tuskegee syphilis study. *Hastings Center Report* 8 (December 1978):21–22.

6. T. W. Murrell. Syphilis in the Negro: Its bearing on the race problem. *American Journal of Dermatology Genito-Urinary Disease* 10 (1906):307.

7. Brandt, Racism, 21–29.

8. Chicago, Il., Mun. Code S36–34 (1966 ed.)

9. Recent studies seem to indicate that even after a needlestick, a health care worker is ordinarily not at high risk. See E. McCray. Occupational risk of the acquired immunodeficiency syndrome among health care workers. *New England Journal of Medicine* 314 (1986):1127–32. R. L. Stricof and D. L. Morse. HTLV-III/LAV seroconversion following a deep intramuscular needlestick injury. *New England Journal of Medicine* 314 (1986):1115.

10. R. M. Veatch. Autonomy's temporary triumph; and D. Callahan. Autonomy: A moral good, not a moral obsession. *Hastings Center Report* 14 (October 1984):38–42.

11. Veatch, Autonomy's temporary triumph, 39.

12. Callahan, A moral good, 42.

13. Quoted in D. R. Hopkins. *Princes and Peasants: Smallpox in History*. Chicago: University of Chicago Press, 1983, p. 86.

14. M. Callen and R. Berkowitz. We know who we are. *New York Native* (November 8, 1982):29.

15. Veatch, Autonomy's temporary triumph, 38.

16. A. M. Hardy et al. The economic impact of the first 10,000 cases of acquired immunodeficiency syndrome in the United States. *Journal of the American Medical Association* 255 (1986):210.

17. Ibid.

18. WHO. Preamble to the Constitution of the World Health Organization, 1946.

19. A. M. Brandt. *No Magic Bullet: A Social History of Venereal Disease in the United States since 1880*. New York: Oxford University Press, 1985, pp. 174–86 and Appendix.

20. F. M. Burnet and D. O. White. *Natural History of Infectious Disease*. 4th ed. Cambridge, UK: Cambridge University Press, 1972, pp. 158–59.

21. For this point, I am indebted to discussions with Steven Miles, M.D.

22. Hopkins, *Princes*, 9–13.

23. J. Goodfield. The last wild virus. In *Quest for the Killers*, J. Goodfield. ed. Cambridge, MA: Birkhauser Boston, 1985, pp. 191–244.

24. Hopkins, *Princes*, 9–13 and passim.

25. 21 U.S.C. S 1175.

26. See, for example, R. F. Boruch and J. S. Cecil. *Assuring the Confidentiality of Social Research Data*. Philadelphia: University of Pennsylvania Press, 1979.

27. Murrell, Syphilis.

# 15 QUARANTINE IN THE AIDS EPIDEMIC

*Timothy F. Murphy*

It is in the nature of epidemics to awaken our worst fears that not only particular individuals will fall victim to a disease but that an entire society may be mortally threatened. The United States, both in its colonial past and its democratic republic, has often been at the mercy of epidemics: Smallpox in Boston in 1721,[1] yellow fever in Philadelphia in 1793 and again in New Orleans in 1853,[2] and the polio epidemic of this century are among the epidemics that have prefigured the medical, social, and ethical issues being raised in today's AIDS epidemic. In fact, some of the issues are identical.

For example, consider Philadelphia's yellow fever epidemic of 1793. Partners and family members deserted one another out of fear of contracting the disease, and other diseases were all but forgotten in the war against the fever. Foreigners were blamed for carrying the disease to the native population; doors were locked against lodgers and their possessions removed; people were afraid to shake hands, churches called days of prayer, and charitable societies raised money to combat the disease and care for the afflicted. Those feared to have the disease were excluded from public places while some individuals with the disease buried themselves in the pleasures of anonymous flesh. Doctors carried on heated disputes about the cause of the disease, experiments of bizarre and grotesque kinds were tried as therapies of the last resort, and government officials consulted daily with medical authorities. Even President George Washington stayed away from the nation's capital as long as he in good conscience could.[3] These avoidances, exclusions, precautions, and efforts all have their parallels in the contemporary attempt to prevent the spread of AIDS.

## ON QUARANTINES

Happily, the yellow fever epidemic in Philadelphia ended when the season of the mosquitoes was ended by the coming of winter. Unfortunately, the AIDS epidemic will not abate without the direct intervention of human beings on an unprecedented scale of complexity and cost. The nature of these interventions is a matter of public debate. It is generally agreed that scientific and biomedical research is a sine qua non in the prevention and cure of this disease. However, there are other, more disputed approaches, quarantines among them, that do not enjoy the luxury of general agreement. Thus far, no red flags saying "God have mercy on this house" have been hoisted over AIDS patients' homes, as was done in Boston's 1721 smallpox epidemic.[4] But other measures equally dramatic have been suggested or at least raised "for public consideration." One may find proposals along these lines on the op-ed pages of many newspapers, in the motions of some state legislators, and in privately stated opinions. There is a strong inclination to consider the question of quarantine as the number of AIDS diagnoses continues to climb without apparent end in sight. I would like to review some proposed quarantine measures and actual exclusionary measures and examine their practical and moral justifications. I will claim that there is neither practical nor moral justification for general confinements undertaken in the name of preventing the spread of AIDS, although certain exclusions have some justification.

Quarantine is classically defined as a period or place of isolation imposed to keep contagious diseases, insects, or pests from proliferating. The term may also be used in a political sense, that is, persons may be confined to contain their ideas or actions. Quarantining is a very ancient notion. In the Old Testament one may find quarantine measures of various kinds. Perhaps the most famous of these is the quarantine of the leper: "A man infected with leprosy must wear his clothing torn and his hair disordered; he must shield his upper lip and cry, 'unclean, unclean.' As long as the disease lasts he must be unclean, and therefore he must live apart; he must live outside the camp" (Leviticus 13:45–46). In our own time, the restraint of communicable disease by quarantine is not without historical precedent. In one famous episode, Mary Mallon, a New York City cook, was committed to jail in 1915 although she had committed no crime. Her incarceration was entirely legal, and she died in jail in 1938, having spent the better part of her adult life there. Mary Mallon, of course, was Typhoid Mary. She had been responsible for some 51 cases of fever, 3 of which ended in death.[5]

Proposals for AIDS quarantine have suggested that inclusion in certain classes of persons or evidence of certain behaviors be grounds for quarantine. In November 1983, a psychiatrist testifying before a State of Texas legislative committee urged that all homosexuals be locked up until such time as they cured themselves of all their medical problems. In September 1985, a British man was ordered into three weeks of mandatory hospital isolation after a diagnosis of AIDS was made.[7] This decision was subsequently reversed not because it was in itself a wrongful action, but because the circumstances of the case were said to no longer warrant quarantine. The fall 1985 announcement by William Curran of Harvard School of Public Health that he was formulating model quarantine laws with a graduated range of confinement measures received much attention in the public press. James Mason, director of the Centers for Disease Control, was also quoted as saying that "in the absence of vaccine and therapy, if we're unable to slow the progress in terms of changing [sexual] behavior and reducing the spread of this virus, society in desperation may come to the conclusion that other, less voluntary measures are necessary."[8]

In several states there has been legislative effort to seek authority to quarantine AIDS patients, either all, as a general class, or merely those who are regarded as posing a specific public health threat.[9] One of the most provocative quarantine proposals thus far publicly stated has been that of Vernon Mark of Harvard Medical School. He proposed for "public consideration" a causal link, first of all, between pornography and the spread of AIDS. Secondly, he suggested that it may become necessary to establish a quarantine for "carriers of the AIDS virus who persist in spreading it by irresponsible behavior."[10] He suggested that such persons be confined to an island in Massachusetts Bay that housed a leper colony from 1902 to 1922. Moreover, in order to be able to identify AIDS virus carriers, he suggested mandatory blood testing. In the interests of fairness, he suggested that prior to the enactment of quarantines, a 90-day educational blitz ought to occur, warning of the consequences of continuing to engage in behavior that contributes to the spread of AIDS.

Other proposals have been less radical and have often taken the form of restricting certain people's access to public places and jobs. School districts have wrangled over whether or not students with AIDS should be admitted. In one case, three New York City children were banned from school because their mothers had boyfriends in a high-risk group.[11] For the U.S. military, the Pentagon has authorized various restrictions on duty or even discharge and exclusion from the service depending on the person's disease status and exposure to the presumptive causal virus, HIV (human immunodeficiency virus). The increasing use of the HIV antibody test has led some people to decline the test out of fear that its results might someday be used as a means of job exclusion, denial of insurance coverage, or even as a means of identifying people who ought to be quarantined. Indeed, a candidate for the mayor's job in New York City claimed that there ought to be mandatory blood testing and that persons testing positive for the target antibody ought to be denied positions as teachers, doctors, dentists, nurses, food handlers, barbers, beauticians, and, of course, prostitutes.[12]

## PROTECTING THE COMMON GOOD

What all these measures have in common is their proposal of a certain kind of isolation or exclusion undertaken to prevent disease transmission. The language of these proposals suggests that they take their legitimation from concern with serving the public good, the common good, or the public health (all used synonymously). The implicit premise involved here is that there is a common good of all people which no single person or group of people may jeopardize by their actions or illnesses, and that this common good might not only permit but require interventions against the endangering presence or behavior of certain people.

Perhaps the most notorious use in recent history of this kind of logic occurred in the confinement of over 100,000 people, U.S. citizens among them, during World War II. This quarantine is instructive to review. In February 1942, under pressure from a number of sources, President Franklin D. Roosevelt authorized the exclusion of certain individuals, enemy aliens and citizens alike, from strategic military areas, claiming that "the successful prosecution of the war requires every possible protection against espionage and against sabotage to national-defense material, national-defense premises, and national-defense utilities." The confinement of the Japanese was a political quarantine said to be necessary for the preservation of the national well-being. Indeed, the formal report of the U.S. Department of War claimed that some Japanese directly engaged in acts of hostility against the United States or at least made such acts possible. The report claimed, too, that after the evacuation of the Japanese to the interior, away from their "suspicious proximity" to regions of considerable strategic importance, such acts of hostility never occurred again.[13]

The logic of this kind of quarantine has many parallels with the kinds of quarantine measures being suggested for controlling the spread of AIDS. In the name of national medical defense one might want to proscribe certain individuals as enemy aliens, deny them access to certain areas or occupations, or even ultimately confine them in the kinds of camps in which the Japanese lived.

Critics of the Japanese internment, however, have been vocal in denying the legitimacy or the efficacy of the confinement measures. For example, one economist has reported that the entire venture cost hundreds of millions of 1940 dollars, money essentially wasted since increased protection of strategic locations would have cost far less and been equally effective against any real or imagined threats from the Japanese in the United States.[14] The social costs of that confinement continue, moreover, to this day. For example, in January 1986, a federal appeals court cleared the way for suits in the amount of $24 billion against the U.S. government as a result of its wrongful actions.[15] In short, the political quarantine of the Japanese was not necessary for the adequate protection of the country, and the costs of the quarantine were out of proportion to its merits. Other measures, equally effective, less burdensome to the Japanese, and less costly would have been preferable to the government-sanctioned, institutionalized suspicion of the entire population of Japanese-Americans.

When one turns to the matter of quarantines for the containment of AIDS, one runs into similar practical difficulties of enormous magnitude. These difficulties may be seen by considering the likely candidates for general confinement:

1. *Confinement of people with AIDS or ARC* (AIDS-related complex). At present this would mean the confinement of some tens of thousands of people, many of whom are in dire need of extensive medical and social support. But this confinement would presumably do little to curb AIDS, since there is no evidence that it is these persons who are generally responsible for the continuing spread of the disease. Indeed, in terms of numbers of people thought to be infected with the causal virus, those with AIDS or ARC represent a tiny percentage of possible carriers. They are the tip of the iceberg. Moreover, they are not known to be more infectious than those merely exposed to the causal virus. Even if one were to identify all those with AIDS or ARC generally, their confinement would not significantly slow down the spread of the disease.

2. *Confinement of everyone infected with HIV.* Estimates of the number of people exposed vary, ranging from 0.5 million to 2 million persons.[16] Presumably this group spreads AIDS more than the group above because its members can be totally unaware of having been exposed and may be completely asymptomatic. To identify those merely exposed, therefore, would require nothing less than mandatory testing of the entire population, since the so-called high-risk groups are fairly invisible and can often remain entirely invisible if they so choose. (Such mandatory testing has been suggested by some.)[17] A second reason that the entire population would have to be tested is that in principle everyone can engage in behavior likely to result in exposure to AIDS, for example, merely receiving a transfusion of blood that is not one's own.[18]

Important practical difficulties attend inclusion of this group for consideration. First, the cost of mandatory, universal testing would be enormous. Second, mandatory, universal testing would also have to be *continual* testing since, like pregnancy tests, it would be accurate only for the day on which the test was made and not for the day following. It would have no power to predict whether a person would subsequently become exposed. Third, there would be some negative reports on blood that is in fact seropositive for the virus. The production of antibodies is not instantaneous but requires some time subsequent to exposure. How long antibody production requires is unknown (but it takes six months in chimpanzees).[19] Fourth, the problem of false negatives also would require that testing be continual, to keep false reports from marring identification efforts. Therefore, if one wanted to institute a quarantine of individuals exposed to the AIDS virus, the plan would necessitate mandatory, universal, and continuous testing of the entire population. This prospect is daunting in its implications for personal rights, economic and social costs, and inevitable failure.

The very likely prospect that carriers of the virus would remain contagious *their entire lives* would mean that lifelong confinement would have to be the order of the day (or at least confinement until such time as some regimen would render them noninfectious). The confinement of up to 2 million people for the whole of their lives is an event I presume no one would ever care see come to pass. The history of infectious diseases, moreover, is such as to suggest that diseases have always been stronger than the quarantine measures taken against them. Even lifetime confinement would be no guarantee that AIDS would be unconditionally halted.

Beyond those issues there are problems associated with testing that might count as evidence against the quarantine of the exposed population. First, there is a debate about whether or not exposure to HIV is a necessary or sufficient cause of AIDS or whether other cofactors are involved. Some have, moreover, made the degree of fallibility of the testing their principal objection to its use. At the present time, too, when public response to AIDS is still evolving, it is unclear just how test results will be used, that is, whether they will become public information or whether anonymity and confidentiality will be protected. If mandatory, universal testing were not adopted and only voluntary testing were available, it is unclear whether people would seek out information that might subsequently be put to detrimental use against them.

The enormity of these difficulties seems to me to be cogent, practical evidence against a general confinement of HIV-seropositive individuals. It is also possible to argue that universal testing is unnecessary in order to control, in a general way, the spread of AIDS. Personal protection, for example, does not require knowing one's sex partner's drug or antibody status. It is enough to assume *that every person with whom one shares a needle or bed has been exposed* and act accordingly. Rather than quarantining individuals who test seropositive it might be enough to educate the public in voluntary measures of self-protection.

3. *Confine those "at risk" for AIDS.* The confinement of people at risk for AIDS is too preposterous to merit consideration, since in principle every person can act so as to be put at risk for AIDS (by visiting a prostitute, having sex with a person whose background is unknown, engaging in particular sexual activities—even, again, agreeing to a transfusion of blood that is not one's own). These kinds of jeopardizing behavior seem to be open to every person. It may very well be the case that some people are more at risk than others, but in principle all of us can put ourselves at risk for the disease. The opposite of high risk is *remote* risk, not *no* risk. Consequently, there is no way to distinguish generally who ought to be brought under the umbrella of quarantine. Is not a continent or monogamous gay man less at risk than a woman who has sexual relations with a number of men over the course of a year? Furthermore, would there be any way to predict generally which individuals would put themselves at risk? It seems to me that insofar as everyone is on the continuum of risk it makes no sense to talk about a quarantine for those supposedly "at risk."

4. *Confine those with AIDS, ARC, or HIV antibody positivity who continue to engage in jeopardizing behavior.* These people have been the object of the calls for quarantine that have been most seriously raised thus far. The difficulty in quarantining individuals of this kind is that it is not possible in advance to determine which infectious individuals are likely to engage in jeopardizing behavior. Moreover, since it is certainly not the case that all sexual relations necessarily expose another person to AIDS, mere evidence that sexual relations took place would not be enough to establish which particular individuals infected their partners. Of course, this does not mean that people cannot and do not act in an objectionable fashion. It is merely to say that there is little support for restricting the life choices of a general class of people because some individuals in that class behave objectionably. One might confine those found to have wittingly put others at risk, but this cannot by itself halt the spread of the disease since presumably only a few of those individuals would ever be known to public authorities. Rather than suggest a quarantine of individuals who do, wittingly and knowingly, persist in objectionable behavior, I think one would do better to construe such behavior as criminal or tortious. I shall return to this point later.

Given the indeterminacies, difficulties, costs, and sheer numbers involved, therefore, it does not seem to me that a case can be made for a general confinement of any of those specific populations. My conclusions thus far are drawn strictly from practical considerations, but I think the argument has moral force as well.

## ETHICAL ARGUMENTS

Generally, moral grounds for intervention in people's choices rest on arguments of (1) diminished autonomy, (2) harm to others, or (3) the disinterested need of the community. Yet it seems to me that none of these grounds, singly or in union, would warrant a general confinement measure in the case of AIDS.

1. *Argument from diminished autonomy.* If a person is incapable of being aware of the significance of his or her actions or is unaware of the implications of the choices made, its often argued that someone else may be better situated to make decisions for that person, even potentially against his or her will. This kind of moral argument cannot be made for intervention against carriers of AIDS or those at risk for AIDS. There is no evidence that such people uniformly suffer from incapacitating or disabling psychical states that, in principle, block an appreciation of the consequences of having anal sex, using dirty drug needles, and so on. No generalizable diminished capacity exists, and to that extent no justification exists for paternalistic quarantine measures.

2. *Argument from harm to others.* Intervention in individual behavior may be said to be justified when that individual's behavior harms other people. Richard Mohr has denied that this kind of moral legitimation could justify restrictions on individual choices, since the harm incurred from participating in at-risk activities is voluntarily incurred (now that blood supplies are generally safe).[20] There are, of course, indirect harms to society, say, in its tax support of public hospitals and so on, but he claims these harms are the costs of maintaining a free society and ought to be borne in the same way that costs of other potentially life-jeopardizing actions are borne. I, too, believe that the notion of harm to others would not in itself legitimate general quarantines if in fact personal autonomy is the kind of unconditional good it is asserted to be. It is, I believe, the case that personal autonomy ought to be respected generally, even if that means that we as a society consent thereby to the indirect spread of AIDS.

This does not mean that no harm befalls anyone. Individuals will be harmed, for example, by partners who lie about having AIDS or having been exposed to its causes. But I think that these risks ought to be borne as the cost of respecting personal autonomy. Conformity to a paradigm of individual responsibility means that individuals and not general classes of people ought to be held responsible for their actions. In this way, a person who continually exposes others to AIDS by engaging in what are considered high-risk activities and who does so without informing his or her partners that he or she has been exposed to the presumptive causes of AIDS might be held criminally or civilly liable for wrongful and reckless endangerment of others. This measure would at least have the merit of debating actual wrongs and not merely feared dangers. I suspect, too, that it would be less expensive in the long run to follow this tactic.

3. *Argument from disinterested need*. I discuss the notion of the community's common good as legitimizing interventions in personal choice by reference to the work of Dan E. Beauchamp.[21] He asserts that from a truly disinterested moral perspective, the distinction between "I" and "you," and between "me" and "them" collapses or conflates into a general concern for community well-being. He argues that we would all, from such a perspective, accept in principle limitations on our choices. His point is this: Limitations or interventions against choices are not inherently objectionable if they aim at sustaining that good in itself, namely, our very lives. That said, Beauchamp also tries to maintain that there are areas of choice that we would not barter away, these being the conditions for achieving our own personal agenda of happiness. I am hard pressed in the case of confinements aimed at AIDS prevention, however, to see whether or not Beauchamp's proposal could resolve the issue. That is, I am unable to tell from his theoretical, communal perspective whether or not such confinement measures would count as a legitimate intervention or whether they would constitute the unacceptable bartering away of areas of choice. I find nothing in his proposals, or those like his, that would show in advance whether quarantines would be acceptable or not. I have similar difficulty with all quarantine proposals justified in the name of the public good, the public health, and so on. That is, I do not believe that these theoretical perspectives adequately distinguish and resolve conflicts between personal and public needs and obligations.

## CONCLUSION

I do not believe that a case can be made for general confinement or quarantine of individuals with AIDS or ARC or of individuals exposed to HIV or at risk for exposure. From a practical point of view, it seems that there is no evidence that such measures, to the extent that they would be possible at all, would in point of fact effectively halt the spread of the disease any more than would a particularly ambitious educational campaign. From a moral point of view, it seems to me that confinement measures would involve an objectionable erosion of personal autonomy. Neither would confinement measures be justified by an appeal to costs, since liberty is costly to begin with. I think, too, that we must come to the realization that the consequences of liberty are perhaps irreducibly tragic.

Some will take exception to my arguments. In October 1985, *Boston Globe* columnist David Wilson wrote an essay, entitled "Time for AIDS Quarantine?" in which he claimed that it was because AIDS has been treated as a "gay issue" that "ideas of quarantine and the adoption of heroic public health measures have been resisted on what might be termed civil liberties grounds."[22] The real issue, he wrote, is the public health, but public health authorities are afraid to raise, let alone support, measures like quarantines "because of a national obsession with minority rights as the ultimate imperative, as first in the national hierarchy of values." Therefore, to the detriment of the common good, "heroic public measures to curtail the spread of contamination are virtually ruled out." Similarly, the *Washington Post* ran a column by neurologist Richard Restak in which he lamented the fact that the public identified with the gay minority with AIDS rather than with people at risk for it.[23]

These kinds of views are lamentable for several reasons. First, the authors of these opinions seem to take AIDS as objectionable only to the extent that it appears to endanger the public at large (that is, the groups they belong to) or that it might cost them tax monies they would prefer spent otherwise or uncollected. This would account for the reason, when the disease appeared confined to gay men and drug users, that these same authors *did not* write columns urging that for the sake of protecting other gay men and drug users quarantines ought to be seriously considered. Second, it is certainly not the case, as Restak claims, that society itself is threatened with extinction. The extinction of society per se would require a much more communicable disease than AIDS is known to be. Third, there seems to be a badly organized hierarchy of moral imperatives involved in these kinds of views. One wonders why the search for a cure for AIDS and a preventive vaccine is not heralded as the "heroic measure" to be taken in stopping the disease. One wonders, too, why there is no criticism of governmental policies that contribute to the spread of AIDS by inaction or censorship of educational materials.

I suspect that major newspapers in Boston and Washington can run such columns because the disease AIDS was and still is seen as a disease of "the Other," people already beyond the pale of society. As a result, the confinement of people already outside the mainstream of society requires little leap in moral logic. Quarantine proposals are of a piece with already existing patterns of social exclusion of gay men and other so-called risk groups. To that extent, emphasis on quarantines could only reinforce already existing prejudices. Moral priority ought to be given to curative and prophylactic measures that would solve the moral dilemmas of AIDS, not to quarantines and exclusions that would only generate irreducible conflicts. In many respects, I see this kind of moral priority as a matter of simple decency, as a matter of repaying the already wronged.

This *does not mean* that action cannot be taken against particular individuals who have demonstrably harmed or who wrongfully expose others to a high degree of risk. These claims do not mean that certain individuals cannot be excluded from schools or occupations if there is evidence that their presence or behavior would be directly harmful. Exclusion is not confinement, and to the extent that exclusion is linked with protection from demonstrable, direct, involuntarily incurred harm there is greater moral justification for it. Hospital ward quarantines, too, to the extent that their purpose is curative rather than merely exclusionary, would also seem morally unobjectionable. Nevertheless, one ought to consider exclusions with the same gravity that one would bring to a consideration of quarantines, for they both involve impediments with respect to life choices. Even if certain exclusions may be justifiable in that context, given what is known about the transmission of AIDS[24] and given the moral importance of autonomy, I do not believe that general confinement measures are practically or morally defensible.

## NOTES

1. O. E. Wilson. *A Destroying Angel*. Boston: Houghton Mifflin, 1974.
2. J. Duffy. *Sword of Pestilence*. Baton Rouge: Louisiana State University, 1966.
3. J. Powell. *Bring Out Your Dead*. New York: NYT Press, 1973.
4. Wilson, *Destroying Angel*, 44.
5. R. A. Knox. Talk of quarantine resurfaces with fear of AIDS. *Boston Globe* (October 7, 1985):47.
6. A. M. Brandt. *No Magic Bullet*. New York: Oxford University Press, 1985, p. 187.
7. Detaining patients with AIDS. *British Medical Journal* 291 (1985):1102.
8. Knox, Talk of Quarantine, 47.
9. Quarantine bill passes Colorado House; LaRouche club moves for quarantine. *New York Native* (April 14, 1986):8.
10. J. Foreman. Massachusetts neurosurgeon suggests quarantine for AIDS carriers. *Boston Globe* (November 21, 1986):30.
11. AIDS and civil rights. *Boston Globe* (October 6, 1985):A6.
12. Ibid.
13. U.S. War Department. *Japanese Evacuation from the West Coast*. Washington, D.C.: U.S. Government Printing Office, 1942, pp. 2–27.
14. L. J. Arrington. *The Price of Prejudice*. Logan, Utah: Faculty Association, Utah State University, 1962.
15. D. Shannon. Rights of war internees upheld. *Boston Globe* (January 22, 1986):3.
16. J. W. Curran et al. The epidemiology of AIDS: Current status and future projects. *Science* 229 (1985):1352–57.
17. R. A. Knox. Medical editor calls for mandatory AIDS tests. *Boston Globe* (April 4, 1986):3.
18. P. Boffey. Panel disagrees over AIDS risk. *New York Times* (October 4, 1985): A16.
19. J. J. Goedert and W. A. Blattner. The epidemiology of AIDS and related conditions. In *AIDS*. ed. V. T. DeVita, S. Hellman, and S. A. Rosenberg. Philadelphia: Lippincott, 1985, p. 22.

20. R. Mohr. Of deathbeds and quarantines: AIDS funding, gay life, and state coercion. *Raritan* 6 (1986):1.

21. D. E. Beauchamp. Public health and individual liberty. *Annual Review of Public Health* 1 (1980):121–36.

22. D. B. Wilson. Time for AIDS quarantine? *Boston Globe* (October 8, 1985):19.

23. R. Restak. Worry about survival of society first, then AIDS victims' rights. *Washington Post* (September 8, 1985):C1, C4.

24. M. Sande. Transmission of AIDS: the case against casual contagion. *New England Journal of Medicine* 314 (1986):380–82.

# 16 HEALTH CARE PROFESSIONALS AND THE POTENTIAL FOR IATROGENIC TRANSMISSION OF AIDS: AN ETHICAL ANALYSIS

*Jacqueline J. Glover and Edward C. Starkeson*

Mandatory screening of health care workers for exposure to the AIDS virus has been advocated by legislators in a number of states.[1] Various organizations within the medical community, including the American Association of Medical Colleges and the American Hospital Association, have also debated policies regarding health professionals and AIDS. This concern over AIDS in health care providers stems from the occupational exposure they have to the AIDS virus and the possibility that they will themselves contract AIDS and spread it to other patients. The known epidemiology of AIDS suggests that it may be transmitted in a manner remarkably like that of hepatitis B virus (HBV).[2] Individuals at risk for HBV infection and transmission through occupational exposure may be at similarly elevated risk for infection by and transmission of the AIDS virus. Physicians and other health care professionals have unique ethical obligations that include the duty to warn patients of potential harm and the duty to take reasonable measures to reduce the opportunity for iatrogenic transmission of disease. Thus, in the urgent effort to control the spread of this "newest epidemic," the health care professions have been identified as a likely place to take action.

In this chapter we argue that mandatory screening, disclosure, and isolation of health care professionals are not ethically required. What is required for health care professionals is to follow barrier techniques recommended by the Centers for Disease Control (CDC) and to take an active role in educating the medical community and the general public about AIDS. We argue that, since the risks of iatrogenic transmission are low and can be further reduced by certain barrier techniques, the harms to individual health care professionals and to the public are too great to warrant mandatory screening, disclosure, and isolation.

The chapter begins with a discussion of the patient-professional relationship as a framework for ethical analysis. The next section discusses the risks of iatrogenic transmission. These two sections will then serve as a basis for the analysis of four questions regarding the health care professional's obligation to discover HIV (human immunodeficiency virus) antibody status, disclose exposure, or withdraw from patient contact.

## THE PATIENT-PROFESSIONAL RELATIONSHIP

Underlying the obligations of health care professionals is the fiduciary relationship they share with patients in the effort to promote health and well-being. The term "fiduciary" refers to the confidence or trust that is a necessary component of this relationship. In promoting this trust, health professionals have a special obligation not to harm patients. This is reflected in the often quoted phrase from later interpretations of the Hippocratic oath, *primum non nocere*—"first of all, do no harm." Patients may not always expect benefit from the fallible medical arts, but they certainly do expect their physicians not to intentionally cause them harm. Physicians, and other health care professionals, have a unique knowledge that obligates them to disclose voluntarily the problems with their services.[3]

Of course, patients also acknowledge that the medical technologies themselves may include a certain risk of harm. What is required for a trusting relationship is not that there be no risks, but that health care professionals responsibly reduce these risks and also adequately inform patients about them. Professionals must respect the patient's individual assessment and choice regarding acceptable risks.

In order for these obligations to apply to the case of health care professionals with AIDS or a positive HIV antibody test, two assumptions must hold true. First, there must be real iatrogenic harm to be expected from seropositive or AIDS-diagnosed professionals working with patients. Closely associated with this, there must be a high enough risk of harm to patients that disclosure is required.

Regarding the first assumption: Even though contracting AIDS is most certainly a harm to those who do, it is a relevant harm in this case only if professionals will, in fact, transmit the disease. The principle of nonmaleficence (not harming) applies only if there are harms to be avoided. And as we will see later, it is wrong to falsely promote nonmaleficence if other important values are sacrificed. At the very least, if other important values are at stake, then the evidence that there are harms to be avoided must be very certain.

This idea of certainty or probability is also associated with the second assumption concerning disclosure of risk. Are health care professionals obligated to disclose *any* risk of iatrogenic harm? First of all, how do we go about measuring risk? One source has suggested that we consider such factors as the probability, imminence, and magnitude of harm as well as the effectiveness of intervention.[4] If we consider only the last two criteria, the risk certainly seems very high, given that AIDS is fatal and effective interventions do not exist. But if we consider the first two criteria, the risk is very low. Compared with the risk that a spouse will contract gonorrhea from an infected partner, the risk that a patient will contract AIDS from his or her doctor through medical procedures is very low. But again, how low is low enough, given the health professional's unique obligations of truth telling and disclosure?

We agree with the predominant view in the ethics literature that the presumption is always in favor of disclosure unless a strong case can be made against it. We think a strong case can be made on the basis that disclosure does not contribute to patient decision making and would cause great harm.

A recent discussion of disclosure in the context of informed consent, by the President's Commission for the Study of Ethical Problems in Medicine and Biomedical and Behavioral Research, warns against a preoccupation with risks.[5] The reason information is provided is to promote patient decision making. But crowding essential information germane to the choice with *highly unlikely* risks of harm does not do so. Moreover, in attempting to determine what risks are high enough to mandate disclosure, one should consider the harms that can come from disclosure itself. The commission report warns against the abuse of such therapeutic witholding of information, but does allow for it "when the harm . . . is both highly probable and seriously disproportionate to the affront to self-determination."[6] The presumption is always in favor of disclosure. Yet a strong argument can be made that the harms associated with disclosure of professional HIV seropositivity or infection are disproportionate to the questionable benefit to patient decision making.

Such harms include the very likely restriction of the personal liberty and livelihood of health care professionals, which could also reduce the available supply of trained health care professionals who are experienced with AIDS. This could compromise the availability of care for patients with AIDS. Such disclosure could also undermine the trust in the patient-professional relationship. By unduly emphasizing risks it could also promote the fear that presently causes the unwarranted isolation and other abuses of patients with AIDS. This would undercut the educational function of the profession because it might suggest to the public, as well as to the health care community, a greater risk than is actually involved.

## RISK OF THE IATROGENIC TRANSMISSION OF AIDS

The provision of medical care by health care professionals is not a recognized means of transmission of AIDS. Transmission of HIV from health care professionals to patients has not been documented.[7] This may be due to the prolonged latency of the HIV infection or to the relatively short period of time elapsed in studies of exposure. In either case, we are dealing with epidemiological probabilities and cannot say there is no risk, or even accurately quantify what the risk might be. But this does not mean that we have nothing to say about risk. If we adopt the model of HBV, as we do in assuming that health care professionals may be a greater risk than other groups, then we know that there are adequate measures that can be taken to effectively reduce the risk of transmission. Epidemiological studies and the analysis of health care delivery methods have demonstrated conclusively the efficacy of a number of methods that can reduce the risk of transmission of all blood-borne diseases, including infection with HBV and HIV.[8]

CDC recommendations for controlling transmission of HBV from health care professionals to patients include suggestions "that carrier personnel who have not transmitted may continue in any occupation, but . . . gloves should be worn for all patient contact."[9]

Reliance upon the CDC recommendations to prevent transmission of HBV would more than adequately prevent transmission of HIV, since HBV is both hardier and more infectious. According to the current director of CDC, "With respect to transmission in health care and other related settings, the hepatitis B model is a 'worst case' situation. Guidelines that would control hepatitis B transmission will certainly prevent the spread of AIDS."[10]

Thus, recommendations for HIV infection from the CDC enumerate "prudent practices . . . [which] should be used routinely" by caregivers to prevent blood-borne infections. These include the cautious handling and appropriate disposal of sharp implements; the utilization of disposable mouthpieces, resuscitation bags, and ventilation devices; handwashing; and the routine use of barrier techniques, including gloves, and gowns, masks, or eye protection where appropriate to the procedure.[11]

If the HIV pathogen were as easily transmitted through like exposures as HBV and had similar infectivity, pathogenicity, and latency, we would expect to find a significantly higher incidence of HIV infection than has been reported, especially among family members of AIDS patients.[12] Thus, there is adequate evidence to suggest that the risk of iatrogenic transmission of AIDS is very low and even those small risks can be effectively controlled by adherence to recommended infection control procedures.

## GENERAL OBLIGATIONS TO DISCLOSE

The first question we address concerns general obligations to disclose. Should health care professionals who have had contact with persons with AIDS inform subsequent patients of their risk for infection with AIDS as a result of the professional's previous contact? Our answer is no. The potential risk would be impossible to quantify, and disclosure would lead to the harms described earlier. In addition, there is precedent in current medical practice against such general disclosure. We do not expect health care professionals to disclose similar iatrogenic risks of transmitting HBV or resistant bacteria such as *Staphylococcus aureus* or *Pseudomonas*.

## OBLIGATIONS TO SCREEN, THEN DISCLOSE

Even if there is no general obligation to disclose, perhaps there is an individual obligation if more specific information is known. Should all health professionals be screened for the presence of the HIV antibody? Many states currently require testing of health professionals for rubella, tuberculosis, and other diseases. Our answer is again no.

First of all, HIV infection presents unique problems for a screening approach. In a population like health care workers, where the seroprevalence for HIV antibody is low, the positive predictive value of the screen will also be low. Currently available antibody tests will only indicate the presence of antibodies to the AIDS virus (and not, of course, the virus itself or its antigens) to a positive predictive value of approximately 35 percent in the general population.[13] This is due to the high number of false positive test results expected when screening a low-risk population. [Editors' note: Positive predictive value is the percentage of true positives among *all* those who test positive (including false positives). Thus, a positive predictive value of 35 percent indicates that of 100 tests, 65 would yield *falsely* positive results.]

Second, the usefulness of screening is also diminished by practical considerations. How often would health care professionals have to be screened: yearly? monthly? weekly? The patient is not really given useful information if he or she is told that the health care professional was not antibody positive at some earlier time. Subsequent exposure to the virus could occur, and this would, of course, not be reflected in the assessment of risk provided by the earlier test.

Third, such screening is very expensive. The exact cost per seropositive health care professional is impossible to quantify without an accurate estimate of the total number of seropositive health care professionals. But the least expensive screening test costs approximately $20. Considering that there are approximately 3 million health care professionals in the

United States, we would spend about $60 million just for the initial screening.[14] The need to use multiple tests (the positive ELISA test must be confirmed by a Western blot test before one is regarded as seropositive) and to perform multiple screens routinely would add exponentially to the cost. Given the low risk in the first place, the money is more justly allocated elsewhere.

Finally, a precedent is also available for the nondisclosure of individual professional risk. We disclose mortality and morbidity rates, in general, as an average for the procedure as performed by all practitioners, even though a particular professional may vary significantly from the average. Such risks associated with the competence of individual practitioners may, in fact, be much greater than risks of communicable disease. And there are also precedents for the nondisclosure of communicable diseases, including, for example, flu, scarlet fever, or HBV. CDC's recommendations require disclosure by an HBV carrier only if there has been a previous documented transmission.[15]

Since we disagree with those who would advocate mandatory screening, it is apparent we also disagree with the disclosure of screening results. The two issues, discovery and disclosure, are connected. If the risk is considered high enough to disclose information, then an obligation exists to discover one's status. If the risk is high enough to discover, then the information should be disclosed to those who face it.

In sum, our objections to mandatory screening and disclosure are twofold: (1) Screening is not really useful, because it leaves open more questions than it answers. (2) The risk to patients is still not great enough to warrant infringement upon the civil liberties of individual health professionals.

## HEALTH CARE PROFESSIONALS AND NONOCCUPATIONAL EXPOSURE

A third set of questions concerns health care professionals who are exposed to AIDS through other means. The risk of acquiring HIV infection and transmitting the virus through medical procedures may be low, but what of the risk of transmitting HIV acquired elsewhere? Should we screen health care professionals who are more likely to be antibody positive by virtue of nonoccupational exposure?

Mandatory screening of only those health care professionals "likely" to contract AIDS obviously faces serious moral difficulties. First of all, how would we determine whom to screen? We would have to single out those known to be at high risk, including homosexuals, bisexuals, people who frequent prostitutes, IV drug users, and perhaps even all adults with multiple sexual partners. Besides more practical difficulties in determining who has had nonoccupational exposure, there are obvious breeches in confidentiality, other personal liberties, and a great risk of harms such as labeling and loss of livelihood. All this for a very low return. Such screening is definitely undesirable.

Do individual health care professionals at such elevated risk have special obligations to discover their status and then disclose it to patients? Do health care professionals have *unique* obligations to avoid nonoccupational exposure? Underlying these questions is the assumption that health care professionals have such strong obligations to their patients that they must alter their own personal behavior in particular ways. We do not usually regard this to be the case. Consider other health-related habits such as stress reduction, alcohol consumption, smoking, exercise, diet, or weight control. As long as they only affect the physician and not his or her patients, such conditions are not regarded as an ethical issue. This is also the key to the risk of the transmission of AIDS. Screening, disclosure, or the alteration of personal lifestyle on behalf of patients are not necessary, because the provision of medical care by health care professionals is not a recognized means of transmitting HIV. Health care professionals have only the same obligations that we all accept to take appropriate measures to protect themselves and others.

Finally, it might be argued that professional impairment could result from the subtle dementia associated with central nervous system involvement with AIDS or from the significant emotional impact of such a severe chronic illness. Both are possibilities, as they are with terminal cancer, for example. Yet we do not argue categorically that health care professionals cannot practice if they have terminal cancer. Such considerations do argue, however, for a case-by-case consideration of the impairment of individual health care professionals.

## HEALTH CARE PROFESSIONALS WITH AIDS

Should health care professionals diagnosed with AIDS be isolated from direct patient care? Until now we have dealt primarily with screening and disclosure of antibody status. We have rejected both on the grounds that they do not fulfill their intended purpose, risks of iatrogenic transmission are low, and harms of both screening and disclosure are great. But the question now arises whether an actual diagnosis of AIDS alters the assessment.

Even after a confirmed diagnosis of AIDS we do not really know when a person is infectious.[16] And it is possible to transmit HIV while only antibody positive. Under the worst-case scenario, we might assume that some individuals are infectious from the time of exposure through the rest of their lives. This would suggest that we should treat seropositive and AIDS-diagnosed individuals similarly. If there is no obligation to discover antibody status through mandatory screening and no obligation to disclose this information or to alter patient contact on the basis of it, then there is no obligation to disclose or alter patient contact on the basis of an AIDS diagnosis either. To do otherwise is to assume that individuals are more infectious while symptomatic, and there is no evidence to document that.

Additionally, the effects of infection with HIV are widely variable, ranging from an asymptomatic status that can last for more than five years, to the milder symptoms associated with the AIDS-related complex (ARC), to clinical AIDS, where death occurs at a mean point of 18 months to two years after diagnosis. To categorically exclude from practice health care professionals who are HIV positive ignores this variability. Withdrawal from patient contact must be determined on a case-by-case basis, with consideration given to the degree of illness and type of involvement with patients.

We have been dealing with the theoretical risk of transmission drawn from the HBV model even though, unlike HBV, the provision of medical care is not a recognized means of transmitting AIDS. According to the HBV model, the more invasive the procedure and the more contact with blood, the greater the risk of transmission. If we use the HBV model consistently as well, we would recommend only the use of barrier techniques and *not* the isolation of professionals from patient contact. That is what is recommended for prevention of iatrogenic transmission of HBV, and there is considerable evidence to support the successful control of HBV transmission when the recommendations are adhered to.[17]

We will thus take the rather controversial position that AIDS-diagnosed professionals do not need to disclose their status to patients and they need not be isolated from direct patient care. This is based on our belief that the risks are low in the first place and can be controlled by adherence to recommended barrier techniques. One study of a Florida surgeon diagnosed with AIDS supports this conclusion.[18] And as we argued earlier, there are real harms to individual professionals, patients, and the general public that will follow from unnecessary disclosure or isolation.

The most difficult question here, of course, involves the propriety of professionals with AIDS conducting *invasive* medical procedures. Certain invasive procedures, especially surgery, do include the opportunity for blood-to-blood transmission if the professional sustains an accident in spite of gloves. As in other areas of AIDS transmission, more research is needed. At the time of writing, CDC had issued guidelines for preventing transmission of HIV in health care settings involving seropositive health care workers performing noninvasive procedures only,[19] but had withheld recommendations on infection controls in invasive procedures performed by seropositive individuals, pending further discussion and internal review.[20]

Our ignorance of infectivity complicates the question. If we isolate AIDS-diagnosed professionals from invasive procedures where blood-to-blood transmission is likely, then we must also isolate those who are only antibody positive. And then we are obligated to discover who those individuals are. Perhaps we should screen all professionals engaged in *invasive* procedures only. We would, of course, have to define what is meant by invasive. This would seem to be the most conservative approach, given the opportunity for transmission by some health care professionals and their unique obligations not to harm. But we must not forget the very real harms associated with those actions and the lack of evidence that health care professionals, even those who do invasive procedures, will transmit HIV. But perhaps that is the price required by a society unwilling to tolerate even a small number of transmissions from a health care professional to a patient. Such transmission may present too serious a breech of the trust required between professional and patient and between the profession and society. Policy-making bodies should be careful to make informed decisions supported by research, but even then they must walk a thin line between the protection of patients and the unwarranted personal harms to practitioners and the promotion of even greater public fears.

## CONCLUSION

Health care professionals do have *some* unique obligations regarding AIDS. They must religiously adhere to recommended infection control precautions. They also have a higher responsibility to set an example of informed decision making on the basis of accurate information and to promote care and compassion, not fear, among members of the health care community and the general public. And of course, should individual practitioners become too ill to provide the proper level of care to patients, they should withdraw.

One understandable line of argument in favor of barring antibody positive and AIDS-diagnosed health care professionals from performing invasive procedures is the associated public relations value. It would show the public that the health care community is concerned and willing to do *something* about AIDS, even if they are not sure isolation is really necessary. But unless all health care professionals performing invasive procedures are screened, isolating only those cases that happen to come to our attention would merely give the public a false sense of security.

In the end, screening in order to isolate clinicians who are diagnosed with AIDS or seropositive for HIV from invasive procedures may be a compromise health care professionals must accept, especially if it reflects a reasoned policy that does not require the general screening and isolation of all health professionals. Such a compromise may represent a societal judgment about the extreme disvalue of even a few transmissions of AIDS from health care professionals to their patients. Further, society may impose such isolation upon health care professionals if voluntary compliance with reasonable infection control procedures is not achieved. However, it should be recognized that such screening and isolation would not promote public education and would come at a very high price to those individual practitioners sacrificed to public fear. As James Mosley has noted: "It should be recalled that the segregation of lepers was found to be epidemiologically unjustified only after countless lives had been ruined. . . . "[21]

## NOTES

1. *From the State Capitals: Public Health.* November 25, 1985 (Florida); November 11, 1985 (Colorado); December 2, 1985 (General); December 30, 1985 (Colorado); March 3, 1986 (Colorado, Idaho, and Arizona). New Haven, CT: Wakeman/ Wallworth, 1986.

2. Centers for Disease Control (CDC). Recommendations for preventing transmission of infection with human T-lymphotropic virus type III/lymphadenopathy associated virus in the workplace. *Morbidity and Mortality Weekly Report* 34 (1985):682–95. J. O. Mason. Statement on the development of guidelines for the prevention of AIDS transmission in the workplace. *Public Health Reports* 101 (1986):6–8.

3. H. S. Perkins and A. R. Jonsen. Conflicting duties to patients: The case of a sexually active hepatitis B carrier. *Annals of Internal Medicine* 94 (1981):524 (Part I).

4. Ibid.

5. President's Commission for the Study of Ethical Problems in Medicine and Biomedical and Behavioral Research. *Making Health Care Decisions.* Washington, D.C.: U.S. Government Printing Office, 1982, pp. 69–102.

6. Ibid.

7. S. H. Weiss et al. HTLV-III infection among health care workers: Association with needle-stick injuries. *Journal of the American Medical Association* 254 (1985): 2089–93. Weiss et al., Needlestick transmission of HTLV-III from a patient infected in Africa. *Lancet* (December 15, 1984):1376–77. CDC, Recommendations.

8. M. A. Kane and L. A. Lettan. Transmission of HBV from dental personnel to patients. *Journal of the American Dental Association* 110 (1985):634–35. M. S. Favero. Sterilization, disinfection, and antisepsis in the hospital. In *Manual of Clinical Microbiology,* 4th ed. Washington, D.C.: American Society for Microbiology, 1985, pp. 127–37. J. S. Garner and M. S. Favero. Guidelines for handwashing and hospital environmental control. *Morbidity and Mortality Weekly Report* 34 (1985):682–95. S. C. Hadler, et al. An outbreak of hepatitis B in dental practice. *Annals Internal Medicine* 95 (1981):133. A. L. Reingold, et al. Transmission of hepatitis B by an oral surgeon. *Journal of Infectious Disease* 145 (1982):262. J. Ahtone and R. A. Goodman. Hepatitis B and dental personnel: Transmission to patients and prevention issues. *Journal of the American Dental Association* 106 (1983):219–22.

9. Kane and Lettan, Transmission of HBV.

10. CDC, Recommendations. Mason, Development of guidelines.

11. CDC, Recommendations.

12. G. H. Friedland et al. Lack of transmission of HTLV-III infection to house-hold contacts of patients with AIDS or AIDS-related complex with oral candidiasis. *New England Journal of Medicine* 314 (1986):344–49. Centers for Disease Control. Transmission of HTLV-III/LAV from a child to a mother providing health care. *Morbidity and Mortality Weekly Report* 35 (1986):5.

13. M. Kanter. AIDS and testing for AIDS (letter). *Journal of the American Medical Association* 255 (1986):743.

14. Personal verification of test costs at local hospitals and laboratories in the Chicago area.

15. Kane and Lettan, Transmission of HBV.

16. In fact, there is some indirect evidence that AIDS- diagnosed individuals are less likely to be infectious. Blood cultures for HIV are positive less frequently in AIDS patients than in ARC patients or asymptomatic seropositive individuals. Personal communication from Larry Falk, Abbott Labs, Chicago, to John Quinn, Department of Infectious Diseases, Loyola University, Stritch School of Medicine.

17. P. E. Anderson. ADA recommends vaccine, other precautionary methods. *Dental Economics* (September 1983):69–75. Kane and Lettan, Transmission of HBV. Reingold et al., Transmission of hepatitis B. Ahtone and Goodman, Hepatitis B.

18. J. J. Sacks. AIDS in a surgeon (letter). *New England Journal of Medicine* 313 (1986):1017–18.

19. CDC, Recommendations.

20. Mason, Development of guidelines.

21. J. W. Mosley. The HBV carrier—a new kind of leper? *New England Journal of Medicine* 292 (1975): 477–78.

# 17 AIDS: ETHICAL, LEGAL, AND PUBLIC POLICY IMPLICATIONS
*Paul Carrick*

Acquired immunodeficiency syndrome (AIDS) is an alien and frightening contagion currently challenging the full resources of our medical, scientific, and human services communities. Much evidence suggests that it will continue to do so in the months and years ahead.[1] Already it has generated an intense wave of vexing ethical, legal, and public policy questions many of which—like AIDS itself—permit no simple solutions. In taking up the challenge of commenting on some of these questions from the point of view of a philosopher specializing in the medical humanities, I am reminded of the Greek legend of the Hydra. The Hydra was a monstrous, nine-headed creature of gargantuan size that ravaged the country of Argos. When none other than Hercules was sent into battle against the repugnant beast, he discovered that each time he cut off one of its heads, immediately two new heads grew in its place. So, too, in grappling with the ethical and public policy issues we are about to explore, I have a very real sense that I will never lay them comfortably to rest. For, from a public policy standpoint, AIDS possesses not just nine heads, but nine times nine. And it is evident that as soon as one of these Hydra-headed problems is satisfactorily resolved, many more rapidly take its place. Lamentably, there is no end in sight to the diverse ethical and legal dilemmas AIDS is spawning.

## THE CHALLENGE TO SOCIAL POLICY

What, then, are the nine issues I propose to confront? They are only illustrative of the monstrous social implications of this infectious disease. Yet all have been widely reported nationally as countermeasures taken by individuals, institutions, or governmental agencies.[2] The following are the nine countermeasures:

1. Some private employers are firing workers who have AIDS or AIDS-related complex (ARC) or are suspected of being AIDS carriers. More extreme still, a few workers have been terminated for having friends who are dying of AIDS.

2. Some school districts are barring or isolating students with AIDS.

3. The Pentagon has instituted its plan to use blood tests to screen everyone on active military duty for exposure to AIDS.

4. Some private corporations are already poised to screen employees on a selective basis.

5. Several life and health insurance companies are rushing to ban or reduce coverage to groups that appear to be at above-average statistical risk of contracting AIDS (for example, single males).

6. Some cities, notably San Francisco and New York, have closed public bathhouses.

7. At least one city, San Antonio, is threatening AIDS patients with felony charges if they engage in sexually intimate contact.

8. Some public health officials are exploring the legalities of a quarantine of AIDS patients who refuse to modify their sexual behavior.

9. Most public health officials are seeking to discourage women who carry the AIDS virus from having babies.

Even a cursory glance at the Orwellian magnitude of some of these measures, all presumably undertaken to protect the uninfected majority from the comparatively tiny fraction of AIDS victims, at once reveals a fundamental clash between societal and individual rights in a new context. On the one hand, there is the undeniable need to take steps to protect the public against the spread of a lethal, contagious disease. On the other hand, there is a danger that, in the process, male homosexuals and bisexuals, intravenous drug users, and other high-risk groups (such as Haitian immigrants, hemophiliacs, prostitutes) will be unjustifiably singled out for discrimination. If so, cherished rights of personal privacy and individual liberty will very likely be violated.[3]

In the following discussion, the bulk of my attention is devoted to examining individually the first five of the countermeasures listed above. In contrast, the remaining four will be briefly glimpsed as a group in order to establish the precise nature of their collective challenge to our ultimate moral values.

Given that the AIDS virus is not easily spread by all infected individuals, say by a sneeze or by casual contact; given that it does not readily penetrate intact bodily systems and does not last long outside the body; given that the disease appears to be contracted by direct exposure of one's blood stream to the AIDS virus, which is carried in body fluids (predominantly blood and semen)—it is my view that at least the first four of the nine nationally reported AIDS countermeasures listed above are wrongheaded on epidemiological and logical grounds alone.[4] That is, upon reflection they show some ignorance of how the disease is normally transmitted from one person to another.

## FIRING WORKERS

To illustrate, take the first countermeasure, firing AIDS victims or known AIDS carriers from their jobs. Here common sense requires us to ask: How many job settings provide the on-site opportunity for the transfer of the employee's blood or semen into the blood stream of others? Furthermore, and aside from epidemiological considerations, as long as infected employees can carry out their regular duties, aren't employers ultimately hurting themselves by dismissing capable workers who may remain asymptomatic indefinitely?

But suppose infected employees develop ARC or AIDS and become too weak to perform on the job. Isn't it just morally wrong to drop such persons from the payroll and cut them off from the employee sick benefits to which they are entitled? I would argue that it is. For, among other considerations, it violates the respect-for-persons principle. The principle asserts that people have value in and of themselves, despite their possibly poor health, and so should be treated compassionately. The respect-for-persons principle is associated with the eighteenth century German moral philosopher Immanuel Kant. But it is also known as an ethical imperative fully consistent with the Golden Rule, which is enshrined in the religious teachings of both the Old and New Testament.[5]

On the legal front, the U.S. Court of Appeals ruled, in October 1985, that people with contagious diseases were covered by a federal law barring discrimination against the disabled. But unfortunately, this statute applies only to federal contractors and to those businesses receiving federal money.[6] Consequently, I propose that the scope of this eminently humane law be amended as soon as possible to cover *all* sectors of the economy, both public and private, not just governmental clients and their employees. However, wholesale efforts to adopt new forms of federal or state legislation to protect AIDS sufferers are probably not necessary. There is mounting evidence to suggest that in almost all states, laws currently on the books that are designed to protect workers against non-job-related handicaps or disabilities can be effectively utilized to protect the livelihoods of AIDS carriers or patients as well. For example, the Civil Rights Division of Oregon's Bureau of Labor and Industries ruled, in January 1984, that AIDS, ARC, or a positive HIV status would qualify as a handicapping condition under state law. In the following year, the same Oregon bureau adopted the specific policy that adverse employment decisions based "on the mere suggestion" of infection with the AIDS virus would entitle the offended employee to file suit under the Oregon law banning handicap discrimination.[7] Even so, equating AIDS with a handicap is a bold conceptual move. The final outcome of this linguistic maneuver still waits on future legal confrontations in Oregon and elsewhere.

The related countermeasure of firing individuals having friends or close relatives who are AIDS patients is an especially pernicious form of employer hysteria. It is irrational because, given the known facts about AIDS, it commits a version of the logical fallacy called *guilt by association*. However, since, properly speaking, there is really no guilt involved here at all but only praise for those who refuse to abandon their dying friends, this logical mistake should be rechristened the fallacy of *disease by association* when applied to AIDS. It is such a blatantly discriminatory and indefensible practice that it must be identified and corrected at every opportunity.

## BARRING STUDENTS

The second countermeasure on my list of nine items that I deem wrongheaded, and for reasons akin to those just cited, is barring or segregating AIDS-infected students from public schools or colleges. For as long as they can perform their studies and exercise reasonably prudent caution in their personal hygiene, what is the medical point? Again, casual contact does not cause infection. It is also pertinent to note that the U.S. Public Health Service reports that, to date, not a single child has been known to have contracted AIDS in schools or day-care centers.[8]

## MANDATORY SCREENING

It strikes me as wrongheaded for the U.S. military to require the mass screening of everyone on active duty for exposure to AIDS. Given what is known about the disease and the currently imperfect methods of early detection, isn't the mass screening plan overhasty?

First, what will mandatory mass screening accomplish? The Food and Drug Administration–authorized ELISA (ensyme-linked immunosorbent assay) blood test may show that a person is "seropositive." In other words, he or she has been exposed to the HIV virus and has produced an immunological response. But the ELISA test is not, strictly speaking, a test for AIDS.[9] It only detects previous infection and antibody response. The telling point is that it cannot, by itself, predict which infected but nonsymptomatic individuals will eventually develop AIDS. Significantly, at present there exists no screening method that can effectively distinguish between individuals who are infected by the virus but are never going to suffer ARC or AIDS symptoms and those who will eventually develop ARC or AIDS.[10]

Second, the often stressful psychological burdens on patients who are notified of positive test results is now well documented.[11] So if the military goes ahead with its mass screening program, it should at the very least ensure that trained AIDS counselors, nurses, and physicians are readily available to adequately interpret to seropositive subjects the meaning of their test results. Presently, it is unclear whether such a comprehensive counseling program will be put in place, given the added expense. Moreover, what can trained AIDS counselors say with any reliable degree of accuracy to a patient who tests seropositive, in view of the additional thorny problem of occasional false positive test results?[12] Regrettably, medical uncertainty over the precise long-term meaning of these tests represents one of the more commonly overlooked stresses of this malady for patient and caregiver alike.

On balance, as Levine and Bayer point out, "the ELISA test is a good one for its purpose: screening donated blood for antibodies to HIV. It can [also] be a useful tool in epidemiological studies, following large populations to track the course of the virus and determining what, if any, other factors may be associated with ARC or AIDS. . . . "[13] Even so, in my opinion it is far from clear to what sound purpose the mandatory screening program of the military ultimately will be put.[14] Presumably, personnel unlucky enough actually to contract ARC or AIDS would have been identified in due time through diagnostic testing anyway and would have received the appropriate medical attention. Since there is no curative medical intervention for those merely testing positive, it follows that much of the anxiety of AIDS is in the waiting game the disease mercilessly plays.

To its credit, the army is planning to test for seropositivity three times, using the somewhat more reliable and costly Western blot test as the last.[15] It also pledges to carefully follow those shown to be infected by HIV, providing them with whatever medical treatment they may eventually require. Only those who develop the debilitating symptoms of ARC or AIDS will receive a temporary or permanent medical discharge, with follow-up medical treatment continuing. All others will remain on duty but will be reassigned to posts in the United States. Yet the social consequences from this mass screening for the enlistees and career soldiers remains problematical. The army is well aware of this, stating in its official magazine *Soldier*:

[Those] who have the virus may be victimized twice, once by the virus and again by fellow soldiers who may want to avoid them. They may lose friends and self-respect because people have the wrong idea about the disease. Knowledge seems to be the only defense.[16]

Since heterosexual males and females as well as nondrug users may also contract ARC or AIDS or test positive and remain asymptomatic for the rest of their lives, and since homosexuality and drug use are statistically linked to AIDS as well as being grounds for dismissal from the service, clearly there will be extra psychosocial burdens placed on those testing positive in the military.[17]

Physicians and nurses serving in the military may face an especially tough conflict of duty here. Reportedly, some are already divided over what to do if an AIDS patient or carrier admits in confidence to a homosexual or intravenous drug experience. Sharing such confidential information could subject their patient to a dishonorable military discharge. If so, as Aaron Epstein asks, writing in the *Philadelphia Inquirer*, which should take precedence ethically in this situation?[18] Should the physician's traditional *medical* duty to keep patient information confidential override the *military* duty to report known homosexuals and drug users to the proper authorities?[19] Whichever decision is made, it is evident that the mandatory screening program will strain the normal conventions of medical and military ethics to the limit. What's more, unless the strictest procedural rules are adopted and enforced to protect the confidentiality of medical records involving tests of AIDS (especially within the military but also in general, whatever epidemiological studies are undertaken), the admitted ambiguity of much of this screening data could unfairly stigmatize a good many military and civilian careers.

## CORPORATE SCREENING

I have already dealt with military screening programs for AIDS. What about corporate screening? Several of the same preceding comments apply, with relatively minor modifications in the argument, to those U.S. businesses and corporations that are now flirting with the adoption of AIDS screening programs as a condition of employment. In many instances, this could only have an intimidating effect on employee morale. It could also lead to serious abuses of the employee's right to privacy. A much sounder plan, I suggest, would be the initiation of employee health education programs. These could be designed to (1) promote safer sexual practices, (2) clarify the sometimes misleading news reports about AIDS, and (3) quell irrational fears among the so-called worried well. I urge anyone who could serve as a catalyst for such programs in their local community or workplace to take up this important challenge.

So far, I have argued that four AIDS countermeasures—firing employees exposed to AIDS, segregating or banning students from schools, requiring mandatory AIDS screening in the armed forces, and requiring the screening of workers in corporate life—are of questionable value in curbing the spread of the disease on epidemiological grounds alone. In addition, persistent ethical and legal questions, such as respecting persons, defining and protecting the common good of all, preserving medical confidentiality and the right to privacy, preventing capricious employment discrimination based on sexual preferences or ambiguous AIDS test results, and providing equal access to educational and career opportunities for those exposed to AIDS, constitute additional civil liberties concerns that no democratically based society can afford to ignore. On the positive side, it is encouraging to observe that many of these complex and contentious public policy dilemmas are slowly being sorted out. For example, public health, corporate, medical, and educational leaders are starting to work with responsible citizens' groups representing diverse interests and viewpoints. Hence, notwithstanding the criticisms I have focused on above, there is evidence that the initial wave of public hysteria over AIDS is receding. And there is every reason to suppose that policymakers are fundamentally united by the common desire to avert what the nineteenth century English social philosopher John Stuart Mill called "the tyranny of the majority over the minority" in formulating society's response to the AIDS crisis.[20]

## INSURANCE DISCRIMINATION

I base the following guardedly optimistic appraisal in large part on recent developments in the health and life insurance industry, the fifth countermeasure on my list. Underwriters of such policies began in 1985 to try to screen out three types of potentially costly clients: first, individuals who do not test positive for exposure to AIDS but are in a high-risk group statistically for eventually being exposed (such as single males, aged 20 to 49); second, individuals who *do* test positive for the AIDS virus, of whom approximately 10 percent are statistically likely to contract ARC (which may or may not lead to AIDS), or AIDS itself, within the next five to seven years;[21] third, individuals who know they have ARC or AIDS and apply for extra life or health insurance coverage while trying to conceal their true medical condition.[22]

In fairness to the insurance industry, it must be pointed out that AIDS is such a relatively new disease that it has not yet been entered into the actuarial tables that insurers use as a basis for setting their rates. Also, virtually no one, inside the gay community or out, defends the conduct of those individuals who apply for large death benefits, knowing they are stricken. Finally, the insurance industry in the United States is a regulated, profit-making institution. As such, it has a justifiable interest in turning an adequate annual profit.[23] Arguably, it also has a presumptive duty to protect its policyholders and itself from carrying any truly excessive economic losses owing to AIDS claims. (Some new data suggest that $147,000 is spent for hospital care alone for each patient with

AIDS; the cost nationally in terms of hospital fees and lost income for the first 10,000 cases exceeds $6.3 billion).[24]

California and Illinois were the first two states to enact laws specifically prohibiting insurers or others from discriminating on the basis of sexual preference. Nearly all insurance companies, however, have begun asking general questions on their applications about current diagnoses for AIDS.[25] Furthermore, in some cases insurers are requiring applicants to take the ELISA or more rigorous Western blot test to detect the presence of HIV antibodies. So far, only California and Wisconsin have restricted insurance companies' rights to use AIDS blood tests. But regulators in other states, notably New York, are weighing similar restrictions.[26]

The point is that in the wake of civil liberties complaints expressed by the gay community and by some state regulators and in the wake of criticism that those who test positive for the HIV antibody were being unfairly discriminated against, since most would never contract ARC or AIDS, the National Association of Insurance Commissions (the umbrella regulators group) has responded in what appears to be a fair and conscientious way. What it has done is to appoint a task force that will study AIDS testing and make recommendations to the individual states, including the legislatures. Significantly, this task force appears to be broadly based politically, economically, scientifically, and socially: Members will include public health officials, regulators, representatives of the gay community, and insurance executives.[27] Granted, it is too early to say what the final outcome of their recommendations will be on these key issues of fairness, equality, and social justice in the delivery of insurance benefits. But surely this multipartisan effort is a step in the right direction.

## THE CHALLENGE TO ULTIMATE VALUES

As for the remaining four issues introduced initially on my list of nine AIDS countermeasures, considerations of space permit only the briefest mention here. It will be recalled that these items were the closing of bath houses, threatening sexually active ARC or AIDS patients with felony charges (attempted murder), placing such sexually irresponsible patients in forced quarantine, and pressuring women who carry the AIDS virus not to become pregnant. I must confess that, in some respects, these are among the most perplexing and sensitive issues stirring about in the current national debates on AIDS. Let me conclude by suggesting why this is so, from both a historical and philosophical perspective.

What these four countermeasures have in common is that they may fall under, and so qualify for, the application of a time-honored, liberty-limiting principle that is deeply embedded in our Anglo-American legal and philosophical traditions. I am referring to the so-called harm principle. It, too, is associated with the English philosopher, John Stuart Mill.[28] Essentially, the harm principle says that society has no right to limit the acts of an individual citizen unless his or her conduct harms the safety or welfare of others. In view of the lethal nature of AIDS, it is arguable that the individual actions these four remaining countermeasures are designed to discourage constitute forms of conduct so hazardous to the welfare of others that they fully satisfy the harm principle's criterion. It will be recalled, for example, that the U.S. Public Health Service has strongly recommended that those individuals who know they are infected with AIDS avoid the risk of infecting others through any form of *unprotected* sexual intercourse (among other precautions) lest they pass the disease on to their unsuspecting partners. Also, infected women are urged not to become pregnant because of the real risk of transmitting AIDS to their infants.[29]

To be sure, the harm principle must always be carefully weighed against another equally powerful moral principle, namely, the principle of autonomy. This latter Kantian principle asserts the right of each rational person to be self-determining, that is, to make choices without interference.[30] In my view, neither principle is an absolute, standing by itself. Informed discussion and reflection will be required to balance properly the principles within our law and public policy on AIDS.

In sum, given the gravity of the threat of AIDS to public health on the one hand, and the need to protect cherished individual freedoms, on the other, the AIDS dilemma represents a fierce contest between potentially conflicting social and personal values. This contest holds in the balance, I suggest, a Herculean test of our humanity and collective good will. Of the nine AIDS countermeasures under discussion, the first four—firing AIDS employees, banning infected students, carrying out mandatory military screening, and carrying out corporate screening—can be shown to be unwarranted on epidemiological as well as on psychosocial grounds. Insurance discrimination aimed at excluding single males from coverage on the presumption that they may fall into the primary risk group of gay men is objectionable not only because such a policy commits the fallacy of reasoning from "some" to "all." More important, such a policy violates the insurance industry's public duty to provide all clients with the opportunity for sound coverage as determined by a fair, medically informed, and evenly applied actuarial standard.

In addition, the remaining countermeasures—closing bath houses, criminal prosecution, quarantine, and prenatal counseling—were found to be prima facie eligible for possible adoption under the harm principle but not without serious qualification. Namely, it is imperative that *society's legitimate interest* in holding those AIDS patients legally liable for their actions who fail to heed the minimal public health precautions be, at the same time, *constrained* by equally careful attention to the legal rights of due process to those so accused. Otherwise, the prosecutory arm of the state may become overzealous. In my view, the right of due process and related civil liberties are the sturdiest bulwarks our democratic society can provide to assure that the reasonable prerogatives engendered in the ethical principle of autonomy can be exercised by *all* individuals without fear of undue paternalistic encroachment by the state, amidst the growing AIDS crisis in the United States.

## A FINAL POINT

It may be objected that by comparing the lethal mysteries of AIDS to the dreadful, nine-headed Hydra, which imperiled even Hercules in the swamplands of Argos, I have injected into this essay an unnecessary dose of pessimism. Not so. As students of the classics will recall, the persistent Hercules, after experimenting with various battle strategies to no avail, finally felled the deadly creature by applying the medical technique of cautery.[31] He discovered that by searing the necks as he cut off each of the Hydra's heads, no head could resprout to resume its terroristic activities over the townspeople it had long abused. So, in my opinion, the Hydra is a fitting and ultimately optimistic metaphor for AIDS. For while many citizens are now understandably frightened, I have no doubt that this microscopic beast will similarly meet its match in the near future at the hands of our persistent and ingenious medical researchers and the courageous townspeople who consent to work with them.

## NOTES

1. AIDS update. *Harvard Medical School Health Letter*. (November 1985):1–4.
2. L. Fish. AIDS is rising concern. *Philadelphia Inquirer* (December 29, 1985): 1E–2E. AIDS. *Newsweek* (August 12, 1985).
3. A. Epstein. As concern about AIDS increases. *Philadelphia Inquirer* (November 10, 1985):2F.
4. AIDS update, 3.
5. Leviticus 19:18, Matthew 22:37–40. See also I. Kant. *Groundwork of the Metaphysics of Morals*. trans. H. J. Paton. New York: Harper & Row, 1956, Chap. 2. First published 1785.
6. See *Arline v. School Board of Nassau County*, vol. 772, p. 759 (1985), 11th Circuit, and *Fair Employment Practices*, vol. 39, case 9. See also *Vocational Rehabilitation Act of 1973*, secs. 503, 504; *U.S.C.*, vol. 29, sec. 794. My thanks to George Brenza for these and related legal citations.
7. AIDS held to be handicap under Oregon law. *AIDS Policy & Law* 1 (no. 5, 1986):6.
8. U.S. Public Health Service. *AIDS Information Bulletin*. (September 1985):1–4.
9. C. Levine and R. Bayer. Screening blood: Public health and medical uncertainty. *Hastings Center Report* 15 (August 1985):10.

10. AIDS update, 5.

11. B. J. Cassens. Social consequences of the acquired immunodeficiency syndrome. *Annals of Internal Medicine* 103 (1985):768–69.

12. K. Mayer. The epidemiological investigation of AIDS. *Hastings Center Report* 15 (August 1985):13–14.

13. Levine and Bayer, Screening blood, 9.

14. The official justification issued by the U.S. Army includes the following: (1) The strength of our national defense must not be weakened by AIDS; (2) the HTLV-III virus must be kept out of the blood supply, especially under combat conditions, where there is no time to screen donors. In this connection, see D. Steele, AIDS: Attacking the problem. *Soldier* (January 1986):10–11.

15. Ibid., 10.

16. Ibid.

17. The U.S. Public Health Service reports that of the 21,065 confirmed AIDS cases in the United States alone as of May 26, 1986, approximately 73 percent were male homosexuals and 17 percent were intravenous drug users. See also L. Biemiller, AIDS on campus. *Chronicle of Higher Education* (October 2, 1985):40.

18. Epstein, Concern about AIDS, 2F.

19. For a parallel dilemma involving the confidentiality rule in somewhat different medical contexts, see P. Carrick. *Medical Ethics in Antiquity*. Boston: D. Reidel, 1985, p. 181.

20. J. S. Mill. *On Liberty*. ed. G. Himmelfarb. New York: Penguin Books, 1974, Chap. 2. First published 1859.

21. P. M. Boffey. AIDS in the future. *New York Times* (January 14, 1985):1C. [Editors' note: More recent evidence suggests that many, if not most, HIV-infected individuals will eventually develop immune deficiency.]

22. L. Fish. AIDS is rising concern. *Philadelphia Inquirer*. (December 29, 1985): 9E.

23. S. Riesenfeld. Health insurance. In *Encyclopedia of Bioethics*. New York: Free Press, 1978, pp. 638–41.

24. Total AIDS care put at $6.3 billion. (Harrisburg) *Evening News* (January 16, 1985):4A.

25. *California Health and Safety Code*, Chap. 1. 11–12, sec. 199.20ff. Fish, AIDS is rising concern.

26. Wisconsin Act 73, Law 1985, effective Nov 23, 1985, codified in sec. 103.15 under "Restrictions on the use of a test for antibody HTLV-III." See also M. Carrol. Revised bill would limit AIDS test use. *New York Times* (February 24, 1986):B1.

27. Fish, AIDS is rising concern.

28. Mills, *On Liberty*, introduction and p. 9.

29. U.S. Public Health Service, *AIDS Information Bulletin*.

30. Kant, *Groundwork*, Chap. 2.

31. E. Hamilton. *Mythology*. New York: Mentor, 1969, p. 164.

# 18 COERCIVE AND VOLUNTARY POLICIES IN THE AIDS EPIDEMIC

*Andrew R. Moss*

As I write, a wave of proposals for compulsory screening for AIDS virus infection appears to have begun. The precedent for compulsory screening was set by the U.S. Army and supported by William Buckley in the *New York Times*.[1] Now, different, sometimes confusing screening proposals are emerging from various quarters, and merging in the public mind with the much more radical and politically motivated proposals for quarantining risk groups.

I think that widespread compulsory screening will not be useful in ending the AIDS epidemic and may lead us in a very dangerous direction. But I also think that compulsory screening proposals reflect the failure of the public health constituency to implement what I would call an aggressive *voluntary* policy for stopping the epidemic, as opposed to what I will define as a coercive policy. I want to propose that if you are against the use of coercive methods in dealing with the AIDS epidemic, then you have a moral responsibility to make effective use of voluntary methods. I am also going to suggest that there is an irrationality in many screening proposals that are aimed, overtly or covertly, at homosexual men. If the main driving force behind the coercive approach to AIDS is the desire to prevent the spread of the epidemic into the general heterosexual population, then an approach aimed at gay men is misconceived because the main avenue of spread is from intravenous drug users, not from homosexual men. The fact that coercive proposals often *are* aimed at homosexual men suggests to me that the coercive approach is a fantasy solution to the problem of the spread of AIDS.

What I mean by a coercive policy is one that restricts individual liberties to achieve public health goals. I would include limitations of sexual freedom such as closing or regulating bathhouses, compulsory use of the antibody screening test, registration of persons seropositive for the AIDS antibody, listing of risk groups, punishment for sexual activity, and quarantine. What I mean by a voluntary policy is one that makes primary use of public education and uncoerced use of the screening test.

When I look at my list of coercive methods I realize that I was personally in favor of closing the gay bathhouses in San Francisco and that I believe that both compulsory testing and quarantine are inevitable in at least some situations—for example (as has been proposed in California) when AIDS cases are found in mental hospitals. So I call the approach that I find myself proposing, which is primarily voluntaristic but acknowledges the need for some coercion, an *aggressive voluntary* approach. I want to give some indication of the origins of this approach. The key experience for me has been seeing the queasiness of public authorities in dealing with AIDS in homosexual men, a queasiness that comes from the stigma that attaches to homosexuality.

## STIGMA AND THE POLITICS OF AIDS

Public health in AIDS has been dogged since the beginning of the epidemic by the fact that the epidemic is primarily in homosexual men, that is, in a stigmatized group whose members have been and remain natural scapegoats for a frightened society. Homosexual men have made up about three-quarters of the cases since the epidemic started, and this concentration has led to a series of attacks on moral grounds from the right wing—beginning with Jerry Falwell's attack in 1983 and progressing to Doctors against AIDS in 1984, and Lyndon LaRouche's activities in 1985. I think it is important to acknowledge that the kind of moral entrepreneuring with AIDS that the right wing has promoted is not incidental but represents a true strain in U.S. society—the strain that produced Prohibition and later McCarthyism. It is because it is a true strain that one finds the shadow of the concentration camps hovering behind any coercive approach to AIDS. My proposition is this: It is because of this hovering fear, and to prevent the use of homosexual AIDS as a wedge by moral entrepreneurs on the right, that the traditionally liberal public health constituency has reacted in the opposite direction, with a hands-off policy for AIDS in gay men.

Three things became clear during 1983: that AIDS really was a sexually transmitted disease, that it had been spread widely among homosexual men, and that it might spread to heterosexual society in general. When it also became clear that the issue of AIDS could be exploited in a way comparable to the abortion issue by right-wingers, many actors in the public health drama felt that they were hearing sentiments uncomfortably close to the traditional plague libels or blood libels used against the Jews. The fear of strengthening these sentiments, of giving ammunition to the libelers, has clearly inhibited many statements by public health agencies and others who have dealt with AIDS and has led many of the actors in the public health drama to minimize the extent of the disease and its association with homosexuality. A characteristic example is Jonathan Lieberson's article in the New York Review of Books,[2] which systematically minimizes the extent of the disease, the probability of progressing from seropositivity to clinical AIDS, and the association between AIDS and homosexuality. A characteristic example from the public health side is the apparent vacillation that Mervyn Silverman, then San Francisco's health director, went through when it became clear that he was going to have to be the first public health official in the United States to regulate gay bathhouses. Among public health officials in general, this fear of strengthening the libelers has led to a general failure to close or regulate bathhouses and sex clubs, to a strong reluctance to use the screening test as a voluntary public health procedure, and to massive prudishness about sexual information. In summary I would suggest that the prospect of the political use of stigmatization by the right wing has led to a reluctance in the generally liberal public health constituency to use coercive or even aggressive methods of any kind. I suspect that it is this failure that is producing a backlash in favor of compulsory methods.

I do not want to minimize the feeling that the gates of the concentration camps are open. Like everybody who has worked through the gay men's epidemic in AIDS, I have often had the uncomfortable feeling that the public discussion of AIDS was poised on a political knife-edge and that the weight of opinion might easily shift towards something like a *pogrom* mentality. We have in fact been lucky with AIDS in at least two ways. First, there was very little spread by bisexuality from homosexual men into the heterosexual population. And second, the risk associated with "casual contact" turned out to be small. In 1983 and 1984, before there was much information on either of these topics, most of us who were making public statements on AIDS were doing so with our fingers crossed behind our backs.

## STIGMA AND THE SCIENCE OF AIDS

At the University of California at San Francisco, we did our first project in AIDS epidemiology—a study of incidence rates in gay neighborhoods of San Francisco—at the end of 1982, just when the epidemic was coming to public consciousness. We did it by identifying neighborhoods of the city in which large numbers of homosexual men lived. This felt, and still feels, like drawing a wall around the ghetto. It led me and others to be extremely paranoid about publishing the results for fear of providing a target—for example, to insurance companies seeking to redline homo-sexual neighborhoods. We did publish the rates, which I think was the correct decision at the time; the insurance companies did not redline the Castro district; and I at least drew a sigh of relief. However, the insurance companies are even now trying to overthrow the bill that prevents them from using the screening test to deny coverage. And I personally have now been subpoenaed by an insurance company trying to deny coverage (to someone who may or may not be in a research study I am conduct-ing) on the grounds of a pre-existing AIDS condition. I will not be at all surprised if some day our 1983 study turns up as part of an insurance company's procedure for getting gay men off their rolls. Does this mean that incidence data should not be published? No, although it does sug-gest that perhaps one needs a better reason for publication than pure professional advancement. What it means is there should be legislation preventing insurance companies from redlining gay neighborhoods.

The point is that the fear of increasing the stigmatization of gay men has a basis in reality, and it attaches to almost any piece of research in AIDS, let alone any public health action, that can be seen as increasing the stigmatization of gay men. This fear can be found, smoldering, in the minds of all AIDS researchers and public health officials in the form of a collection of poorly differentiated anxieties: that insurance companies are just waiting to disenfranchise gay men, that the right wing is going to launch a scapegoating crusade, that the gates of the concentration camps are opening. This collection of anxieties has held public health authori-ties back from a whole range of public health actions that might be seen as increasing stigma, and has therefore polarized debate between a pro-tective public health constituency that is seen as being afraid to act and a victimizing right-wing political constituency that is seen as being morally absolutist. This polarization, it seems to me, is something we want to avoid.

## CLOSING THE BATHS

Closing the baths in San Francisco was the original stigmatizing public health act in the history of AIDS and it was, of course, a symbolic act. Not even the advocates, of whom I was one, believed that closing, or regulating,[3] the baths would have a dramatic effect on the AIDS inci-dence rate in the city. I think that most of us believed, first, that closing the baths would have *some* effect on the incidence rate; second, that the closing made clear that we thought AIDS really *was* a sexually transmit-ted disease; and third, that the closing showed that the authorities really did take the epidemic seriously. Beneath these specifics there was per-haps an underlying stratum of obligation. I suspect that most of us felt that we would have to turn in our badges, as it were, if we did not try to close the baths. Although the responsibility is not formally expressed, there seems to be a kind of "compulsion to prevent" in the public health constituency, which you can feel if you are in a position of power and which is somewhat analogous to the clinician's compulsion to treat. You have got to do something, or why are you wearing that badge?

During the bath-closing debate, which took place in the press, in political circles, and in Mervyn Silverman's office, two things became clear to me. First, a disease's stigmatization of a population does not confer on that population an exemption from coercive public health measures. Preventing homosexual men from being blamed for the AIDS epidemic does not require prohibiting all measures that could reflect adversely on homosexuals. But, second, if a public health official was going to advocate coercive measures that were clearly stigmatizing, then it must be clear that they are advocated for health reasons, not moral-political reasons. I had to distinguish myself from, say, Doctors Against AIDS in Dallas, who were advocating AIDS quarantine measures at that same time. The way to do this, it seemed, was to publicly support and lobby for legislation and regulation that made it impossible, or at least difficult, to use public health actions for discriminatory purposes. In California that meant supporting the Agnos bill, which was then in committee and which made it illegal to use the antibody test without consent or in order to limit insurance coverage. Therefore, I went up to Sacramento and testified before the Health Committee of the California Assembly in support of the bill.

The second thing I learned was how much I disliked having to use what was perceived as a coercive intervention, and how much I did not want to have to do it in the future—much less use more seriously coercive interventions like registration and compulsory testing. It became clear to me during what eventually became the bathhouse regulation process that if you do not want to make homosexual men scapegoats through the use of overtly coercive policies—either because you don't think the response is appropriate or because you think the dangers outweigh the benefits—then you absolutely *must* take responsibility for designing and launching voluntary methods that work. At the time that meant pushing hard for the development of "alternative test sites," where anyone could get the antibody test done anonymously along with the follow-up that this voluntary screening entails. I supported that and was described at the time as being the "Nazi" (relatively speaking, I suppose) among the group of researchers and physicians who made up the public health constituency.[4]

In summary, I learned two lessons as a result of being forced by the bathhouse-regulation process into the uncomfortable position of publicly advocating sexual regulation. The first thing I learned was that the way to offset the stigmatizing effect of coercive public health measures is to operate politically against the stigmatization. And the second thing I learned was that if it makes you uncomfortable to administer (even mildly) coercive methods to stop or slow down the epidemic, then you had better make sure that there are voluntary methods which work.

Many people in San Francisco reached similar conclusions in 1983–84, and I think it is fair to characterize San Francisco policy in the gay male AIDS epidemic as an aggressively voluntaristic one, with some coercion in the case of the bathhouse regulations. We have pushed hard on publicly funded education, including sexual education; on encouraging, or at least making available, the antibody test; and on supporting the conscious attempt in the gay community to change attitudes and relational styles. I draw some comfort from the fact that the epidemic seems to have stabilized among gay men—that is, the numbers of new cases per month are stabilizing and the seroconversion rate among gay men appears to be down considerably from its peak.[5] At present (my fingers are crossed again) the voluntary approach seems to be paying off. I think we should further encourage the voluntary use of the screening test and keep up the educational pressure. There is a tendency for our public health bureaucracy to sink back into primeval inertia when direct media pressure is removed. If we in San Francisco were to summarize what we did for export (and I think we should export it, along with the AIDS Clinic and the famous San Francisco support services model) I would call it an aggressive voluntarist approach, in which the health authorities did not (quite) shrink from what was seen as coercion when it was necessary, and in which there was a strong offsetting political effort to make it clear that the authorities were committed to a noncoercive overall policy.

## INAPPROPRIATE COERCION

Having made a pitch for aggressive voluntarism, I would now like to look at the other side of the coin, which is the inappropriate use of coercion. This is likely to arise, I suspect, in the other AIDS epidemic, among intravenous drug users. While this second epidemic currently presents a relatively small clinical problem outside the East Coast, it threatens to become a major public health problem. There are two reasons for this. First, new infections may be growing almost as fast among drug users as among homosexual men. Second, it is from intravenous (IV) drug users that AIDS is spreading heterosexually into the general population.

In San Francisco, AIDS in drug users is probably creating almost as many newly infected people right now [1986] as AIDS in gay men. This is because among IV drug users the epidemic is at the beginning of its career, while AIDS in gay men has peaked. There was a 2.0 to 4.6

percent conversion rate in 1985 among seronegative gay men in San Francisco, which translates to between 500 and 1,150 newly infected gay men in that year.[6] While these numbers are shockingly high, they are down from over 2,000 a year at peak (more than 20,000 gay men have been infected in San Francisco in less than ten years), and the numbers are still falling.

Among IV drug users in San Francisco, however, the number newly infected every year is probably rising. There were some 700 seropositive drug users in the city in 1985.[7] If we look at what has happened in New York or in the nation as a whole, or we look at successive studies done in various European countries, we see that AIDS in drug users has generally grown at about the same rate as AIDS in gay men, doubling about once a year in the first years of the epidemic. Hence, drug users may be getting infected in San Francisco at a rate of about 700 a year—about comparable to the rate in homosexual men. But the rate in drug users is going up, while the rate in homosexual men is probably coming down. These numbers say that a sizable fraction of our preventive effort, perhaps close to half, should be in preventing AIDS in drug users. Probably rather similar calculations could be made for any city where the gay male epidemic has matured and the drug use epidemic is just beginning, that is, most U.S. and European cities other than the New York–New Jersey conurbation.

It is *already* true, unfortunately, that most of the heterosexual spread of AIDS is from drug users. The Centers for Disease Control maintains figures on heterosexual transmission, and so far, two-thirds of the heterosexual transmission cases have been from intravenous drug users. It is also true that more than half of all children with AIDS have at least one drug-using parent.[8] While transmission from children is not currently a problem in the United States, the long-run prospect of widespread perinatal transmission is distressing. Finally, almost all seropositive prostitutes so far reported have been intravenous drug users. If what we are worried about is heterosexual spread of AIDS into the general population, then preventing the spread of AIDS among drug users is where the energy should go.

I go through this exercise to make it clear that draconian proposals for dealing with seropositives and which are allegedly intended to protect the heterosexual population are irrational if the subtext is that they are aimed at homosexual men. Even though gay men with AIDS outnumber drug users with AIDS by about four to one, most of the heterosexual spread of AIDS is from the drug users. It is a major index of the irrationality of public thinking on AIDS that until recently there was almost no public health acknowledgment of this situation. A second index of irrationality is that in many state and city governments in the United States, it is easier to discuss quarantining or compulsory screening of homosexual men than legalizing needle use or other policies that recognize that drug users will likely go on shooting drugs, regardless. On the one hand, we are willing to countenance a public discourse about mass screening and quarantining of the wrong population. On the other hand, we can barely discuss one of the few available interventions with the right population.

However, once it becomes clear that the drug-user epidemic is expanding and is responsible for most heterosexual transmission of AIDS, drug users may well be targeted for quarantine or preemptive screening measures. The two public examples of sexual incorrigibility in AIDS so far, one male in Dallas and one female in New Haven, were both intravenous drug users. I suspect that it is here that coercive methods are likely to be proposed, most probably enforced screening in treatment programs, perhaps with some kind of incarceration for recalcitrant seropositives. Perhaps the main danger here is that public health policy, like research funding, is decided in discontinuous lurches in response to media pressure. When federal and state public agencies acknowledge that preventing heterosexual transmission of AIDS means doing something serious about AIDS in drug users, a problem that has been more or less ignored so far, they may be stampeded into coercive action.

But coercive measures in this population will clearly not work, unless it is proposed to find and incarcerate the whole needle-using population of the United States, which on current estimates would roughly double the size of the prison population. What will happen if a coercive approach is taken? It can only be done through treatment programs, and it would probably chase a high proportion of drug users out of the program, thus in the end perhaps finding no more seropositives than we can already find by voluntary methods. Furthermore, the use of any kinds of compulsory methods in treatment programs will raise issues that must be decided in court, which will freeze the development of any voluntary screening. And finally, the public health authorities will lose whatever fragile credibility they have among their clients, so that if coercive methods fail, which they almost certainly will in a population that is *already* outside the law, then what will we do next?

Here, once again, it is important to acknowledge that if one does not want to see coercive methods used one has the responsibility to design a voluntary intervention program that works. I believe that such an intervention should be organized around an intensive, voluntary use of the screening test to find the seropositives—still only in the hundreds in San Francisco—and to work with them intensively, get them into treatment, and at least slow the epidemic down until a vaccine becomes available or the distribution of clean needles is legalized. We have had relatively good success with at least the screening part of this approach in San Francisco; I am not sure what is required to keep those we find to be seropositive in treatment, or to keep them from sharing needles. However, we will not find out until we try.

To end on an optimistic note, I should say that San Francisco and, to some extent, the State of California have been models so far for the use of voluntary policies and that, in gay men at least, the policies seem to have been relatively successful. Much of the credit for this success goes to the gay political lobbies and to some statewide politicians with large gay constituencies. What it comes down to is that AIDS is a political disease. The scope of AIDS politics has now been broadened from a few cities to the country as a whole, and from the narrow public health arena to the whole political process. If we do not want to see the governmental machinery stampeded into inappropriate and destructive coercive policies—policies that may well make voluntary methods impossible—then we have to expand the lessons of the bathhouse regulation to the wider sphere. We in the public health community have to acknowledge that if we do not want coercive methods used, we have a responsibility to design voluntary methods that work.

## NOTES

1. W. F. Buckley, Jr. Crucial steps in combatting the AIDS epidemic: Identify all the carriers. *New York Times* (March 18, 1986):A27.

2. *New York Review of Books* (January 16, 1986).

3. Silverman's eventual strategy was to prohibit what were thought to be risky sexual activities in bathhouses licensed by the city.

4. Similarly, a gay colleague was described as "Dr. Mengele" when he supported the initial vote to regulate the bathhouses. The gay politicians who supported the final regulation were pilloried in the leading gay newspaper under the headline "Their Names Shall Live in Infamy." [Editors' note: This episode is described in detail in R. Shilts. *And the Band Played On: Politics, People, and the AIDS Epidemic*. New York: St. Martin's Press, 1987.]

5. The rate at which new cases were diagnosed was stable at about 65 a month in 1985 and rose slightly to about 75 a month at the beginning of 1986 (G. Rutherford, San Francisco Department of Public Health, personal communication.) This followed a period during 1981–84 when the rate rose almost exponentially. [See A. R. Moss, et al. Incidence of the acquired immunodeficiency syndrome in San Francisco. *Journal of Infectious Disease* 152 (1985):152–161.] The seroconversion rate in the San Francisco General Hospital study was 2 percent per year in randomly selected homosexual men in 1985 (A. R. Moss, unpublished data). The seroconversion rate in the San Francisco Gay Men's Health Study was 4.6 percent (W. Winkelstein, personal communication.)

6. There are about 50,000 homosexual men in San Francisco, and about half of them were seropositive in 1985 (San Francisco General Hospital study, unpublished data, and W. Winkelstein, personal communication). Applying the seroconversion rates given in the text to the 25,000 uninfected men yields the estimate that between 500 and 1,150 men became seropositive in 1985–86.

7. About 10 percent of the treatment population of some 4,000 users and 2–4 percent of the population of about 8,000 users who have never been in treatment. Seropositivity rates are from unpublished data furnished by courtesy of R. Chaisson, Department of Medicine, San Francisco General Hospital. User population estimates are from J. Newmeyer, Haight-Ashbury Free Medical Clinic.

8. Of 273 heterosexual-contact cases reported to the Centers for Disease Control 163 were attributed to IV drug use, and 150 of 277 children with AIDS had at least one drug-using parent, as of April 1986 (A. Hardy, Centers for Disease Control, personal communication).

# FOR FURTHER READING

## BOOKS

Altman, Dennis. *AIDS in the Mind of America*. Garden City, NY: Doubleday, 1986.

Black, David. *The Plague Years: A Chronicle of AIDS, the Epidemic of Our Times*. New York: Simon & Schuster, 1985.

Brandt, Allan. *No Magic Bullet: A Social History of Venereal Disease in the United States Since 1880*, Rev. ed. New York: Oxford University Press, 1987.

Cahalan, Kathleen, ed. *AIDS: Issues in Religion, Ethics, and Health Care (A Park Ridge Bibliography)*. Park Ridge, IL: The Park Ridge Center, 1988.

Cole, Helene, and George Lundberg, eds. *AIDS: From the Beginning*. Chicago: American Medical Association, 1986.

Feldman, Douglas, and Thomas Johnson, eds. *The Social Dimensions of AIDS: Method and Theory*. New York: Praeger, 1986.

Fortunato, John. *AIDS: The Spiritual Dilemma*. San Francisco: Harper & Row, 1987.

Griggs, John, ed. *AIDS: Public Policy Dimensions*. New York: United Hospital Fund of New York, 1987.

Humbar, James, and Robert Almeder, eds. *Biomedical Ethics Reviews: 1989*. AIDS and Ethics. Clifton, NJ: Humana Press, 1989.

Pierce, Christine, and Donald VanDeVeer, eds. *AIDS:Ethics and Publicy Policy*. Belmont, CA: Wadsworth, 1988.

Shilts, Randy. *And the Band Played On: Politics, People and the AIDS Epidemic*. New York: St. Martin's Press, 1987.

## ARTICLES

Bayer, Ronald. "Gays and the Stigma of Bad Blood." *Hastings Center Report* 13 (April 1983):5–7.

_____. "AIDS, Power, and Reason." *Milbank Quarterly* 64 (1986):168–82.

Bayer, Ronald, Carol Levine, and Susan Wolf. "HIV Antibody Screening: An Ethical Framework for Evaluating Proposed Programs." *Journal of the American Medical Association* 256 (1986):1768–74.

Beauchamp, Dan E. "Morality and the Health of the Body Politic." *Hastings Center Report* 16 (December 1986):30–36.

Brandt, Allan. "AIDS: From Social History to Social Policy." *Law, Medicine and Health Care* 14 (1986):231–42.

Conrad, Peter. "The Social Meaning of AIDS." *Social Policy* 17 (1986):51–56.

Eisenberg, Leon. "The Genesis of Fear: AIDS and the Public's Response to Science." *Law, Medicine and Health Care* 14 (1986):243–49.

Emanuel, Ezekiel. "Do Physicians Have an Obligation to Treat Patients with AIDS?" *New England Journal of Medicine 381* (1988):1686–90.

Fox, Daniel. "AIDS and the American Health Polity: The History and Prospects of a Crisis in Authority." *Milbank Quarterly* 64 (1986):7–33.

_____. "From TB to AIDS: Value Conflicts in Reporting Disease." *Hastings Center Report* 16 (December 1986):11–16.

Goldberg, Stephanie. "The Meaning of 'Handicapped'." *American Bar Association Journal* 73 (March 1, 1987):56–61.

Gillet, Grant. "AIDS and Confidentiality." *Journal of Applied Philosophy* 4 (1987): 15–20.

Gostin, L. O., W. J. Curran, and M. Clark. "The Case Against Compulsory Casefinding in Controlling AIDS." *American Journal of Law and Medicine* 12 (1987):7–53.

Jonsen, Albert, Molly Cooke, and Barbara Koenig. "AIDS and Ethics." *Issues in Science and Technology* 2 (1986):56–65.

Kayal, Philip. "'Morals,' Medicine and the AIDS Epidemic." *Journal of Religion and Health* 24 (1985):218–38.

Kelly, J. A., et al. "Stigmatization of AIDS Patients by Physicians." *American Journal of Public Health* 77 (1987):789–91.

Koenig, Barbara. "Ethical and Legal Issues of the AIDS Epidemic." In *Nursing Care of the Patient with AIDS/ARC*. Edited by Angie Lewis. Rockville, MD: Aspen, 1988.

Macklin, Ruth. "Predicting Dangerousness and the Public Health Response to AIDS." *Hastings Center Report* 16 (1986):16–23.

McCombie, S. C. "The Cultural Impact of the 'AIDS' Test: The American Experience." *Social Science and Medicine* 239 (1986):455–59.

Milliken, Nancy, and Ruth Greenblatt. "Ethical Issues of the AIDS Epidemic." In *Medical Ethics: A Guide for Health Professionals*. Edited by John Monagle and David Thomasma. Rockville, MD: Aspen, 1988.

Mills, Michael, Constance Wofsy, and John Mills. "The Acquired Immunodeficiency Syndrome: Infection Control and Public Health Law." *New England Journal of Medicine* 314 (1986):931.

Musto, David. "Quarantine and the Problem of AIDS." *Milbank Quarterly* 64 (1986):97–117.

Pellegrino, Edmund. "Altruism, Self-Interest, and Medical Ethics." *Journal of the American Medical Association* 258 (1987):1924–28.

Purtilo, Ruth, Joseph Sonnabend, and David Purtilo. "Confidentiality, Informed Consent, and Untoward Social Consequences in Research on a 'New Killer Disease' (AIDS)." *Clinical Research* 31 (1983):462–72.

Relman, Arnold, ed., "AIDS: The Emerging Ethical Dilemmas." *Hastings Center Report* 15 (August 1985), Special Supplement.

Rosenberg, Charles. "Disease and Social Order in America: Perceptions and Expectations." *Milbank Quarterly* 64 (1986):34–55.

Spohn, William C. "The Moral Dimensions of AIDS." *Theological Studies* 49 (March 1988):89–109.

Steinbrook, Robert, et al. "Ethical Issues in Caring for Patients with Acquired Immunodeficiency Syndrome." *Annals of Internal Medicine* 103 (1985):787–90.

Zuger, Abigail, and Steven Miles. "Physicians, AIDS, and Occupational Risk: Historic Traditions and Ethical Obligations." *Journal of the American Medical Association* 258 (1987):1924–28.

# INDEX

Mosley, James, 161
Murrell, Thomas, 131–32, 138

nausea and the fear of death, 51
*Night Sweat* [play], 42
nomenclature, 3–11, 25–26
nonoccupational exposure of health
care providers, 157–58
*The Normal Heart* [Kramer], 42–43, 47,
48–49

obligations. *See* Duty
*One* [play], 42
Oppenheim, P., 25
Oroszlan, Stephen, 10
otherness metaphor, 37–39

paternalism, 112–13, 129, 134–35, 147
patients: advance directives of, 94–99;
competent, 86, 87–88, 96; decision
making by, 86–92, 94–99; fear of
exposure to, 74–75; gender as a
factor in caring for, 78–79; health
care providers relationship with,
153–54; identification with, 76–77,
83, 86; incompetent, 91–92, 96–97,
113–15; obligations to, 72–84;
refusals to care for, 74–75, 80, 81;
violent, 109, 112–13. *See also* caring
for patients
Perloff, Joseph, 33
philosophy of revolt, 59
physicians. *See* health care providers
physicochemistry, 14
*The Plague* [Camus], 38, 57–59
plagues, 50, 51, 54–59, 66. *See also*
epidemic
plays about AIDS, 42–49
pneumocystis pneumonia, 54, 87–88,
95–96, 105
polio, 66, 140
political quarantine, 36–37, 143–44
politics of AIDS, 19, 174, 175–76, 182
pornography, 142
positivistic philosophy, 18
precautions, 79–80, 126, 155, 159. *See
also name of specific precaution*
pregnant women, 164, 170–72

President's Commission for the Study
of Ethical Problems in Medicine and
Biomedical and Behavioral Research,
154
privacy/freedom, 119–27. *See also*
autonomy
promiscuity, 16–17, 33–34, 44, 48–49,
146. *See also* sexual practices
prostitution, 126, 180
protest art, 43–45
prudent practices, 155
psychological burdens of positive
screening, 167–68
psychological effects of nomenclature,
6
psychotherapists, 109, 112–15
public health measures. *See* public
policies
public policies: aggressive voluntary,
175, 177–79; AIDS as a challenge to,
163–65; coercive, 120, 174–82; and
contagious disease, 129; and
decision making, 120–27; and
discrimination, 178; and divisiveness
in society, 176–77; and drug users,
120, 179–81; and ethics, 165–66; and
fear, 175–76; and gay men, 120; and
the harm principle, 170–71; inappropriate, 179–82; and the mentally ill,
125; and privacy/freedom, 119–27;
restrictive, 119–27; and sexual
practices, 170–72, 175; and stigma,
120, 178–79; voluntary, 174–82. *See
also name of specific type of measure*
punishment, 32–34, 39, 55, 64, 69, 91,
131–32, 175

quality of life, 103–4
quarantine: advocates for, 178; of ARC
carriers, 144; and autonomy, 147;
and the common good, 136, 143–46,
148–49; conditions for, 125; and
contagious disease, 125, 131, 141;
and costs, 143–44, 149; definition of,
141; and discrimination, 129, 149;
and divisiveness in society, 149; and
drug users, 149, 181; effects of, 144,
145, 148; and epidemic, 140–50; and

# CONTRIBUTORS

**JANA L. ARMSTRONG, M.PHIL.,** Jacob K. Javits Research Fellow, Department of Anthropology, University of Kansas, Lawrence, Kansas

**JOSEPH CADY, PH.D.,** Visiting Professor (Literature), Division of Medical Humanities, School of Medicine and Dentistry, University of Rochester, Rochester, New York

**PAUL CARRICK, PH.D.,** Professor of Philosophy, Harrisburg Area Community College, Harrisburg, Pennsylvania

**MOLLY COOKE, M.D.,** Assistant Clinical Professor of Medicine, San Francisco General Hospital, University of California–San Francisco, San Francisco, California

**MARY ANN GARDELL CUTTER, PH.D.,** Adjunct Assistant Professor, Department of Philosophy, University of Colorado–Denver, Denver, Colorado

**JACQUELINE J. GLOVER, PH.D.,** Instructor, Department of Health Care Sciences, The George Washington University Medical Center, Washington, D.C.

**KATHRYN MONTGOMERY HUNTER, PH.D.,** Co-Director, Program in Ethics and Human Values, Northwestern University Medical School, Chicago, Illinois

**ALBERT R. JONSEN, PH.D.,** Professor of Ethics in Medicine and Chair, Department of Biomedical History and Ethics, School of Medicine, University of Washington, Seattle, Washington

**ERIC T. JUENGST, PH.D.,** Assistant Professor of Humanities (Philosophy), Department of Humanities, Pennsylvania State University College of Medicine, Milton S. Hershey Medical Center, Hershey, Pennsylvania

**BARBARA A. KOENIG, R.N., PH.D.,** Nursing Education Coordinator, AIDS Professional Education Project *and* Adjunct Lecturer, Division of Medical Ethics, University of California–San Francisco, San Francisco, California

**BERNARD LO, M.D.,** Associate Professor of Medicine, School of Medicine, University of California–San Francisco, San Francisco, California

**ERICH H. LOEWY, M.D.,** Assistant Professor of Medicine, University of Illinois College of Medicine, Peoria, Illinois, *and* Assistant Professor of Humanities (Ethics), University of Illinois, Chicago, Illinois

**RAY E. MOSELEY, PH.D.,** Director, Medical Humanities Program, Department of Community Health and Family Medicine, University of Florida College of Medicine, Gainesville, Florida

**JOHN C. MOSKOP, PH.D.,** Associate Professor of Medical Humanities, East Carolina University School of Medicine, Greenville, North Carolina

**ANDREW R. MOSS, PH.D.,** Associate Professor in Residence, Department of Epidemiology and International Health, School of Medicine, University of California–San Francisco, San Francisco, California

**JULIEN S. MURPHY, PH.D.,** Assistant Professor of Philosophy, Department of Philosophy, University of Southern Maine, Portland, Maine

**TIMOTHY F. MURPHY, PH.D.,** Assistant Professor of Philosophy, Boston University, Boston, Massachusetts

**LAWRENCE J. NELSON, PH.D., J.D.,** Bioethics Consultation Group, Berkeley, California, *and* Adjunct Lecturer, Division of Medical Ethics, University of California–San Francisco, San Francisco, California

**JUDITH WILSON ROSS, PH.D.,** Associate Director, Program in Medical Ethics, University of California–Los Angeles, Los Angeles, California, *and* Associate, Center for Bioethics, St. Joseph Health System, Orange, California

**EDWARD C. STARKESON, M.P.H.,** School of Public Health, University of Illinois, Chicago, Illinois

**CAROL A. TAUER, PH.D.,** Professor of Philosophy, Department of Philosophy, The College of St. Catherine, St. Paul, Minnesota

**HAROLD E. VARMUS, M.D.,** American Cancer Society Professor of Molecular Virology, Department of Microbiology and Immunology, University of California–San Francisco, San Francisco, California

**WILLIAM J. WINSLADE, PH.D., J.D.,** Professor of Medical Jurisprudence and Psychiatry, Institute for the Medical Humanities, University of Texas Medical Branch, Galveston, Texas